THE MODERN MAN

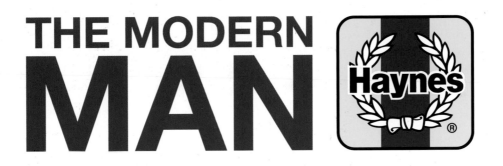

To the women who made a man of me:
Catherine, Francesca and Luciana.

Richard Hutt has asserted his right to be identified
as the author of this work.

First published in November 2017

British Library Cataloguing in Publication Data
A catalogue record for this book is available
from the British Library.

ISBN 978 1 78521 140 9

Library of Congress catalog card no. 2017933527

Published by Haynes Publishing,
Sparkford, Yeovil, Somerset BA22 7JJ, UK
Tel: 01963 440635
Int. tel: +44 1963 440635
Website: www.haynes.com

Haynes North America Inc.
861 Lawrence Drive, Newbury Park,
California 91320, USA

Designed by Richard Parsons

Printed and bound in Malaysia

A note on gender and sexuality: this book makes no assumptions as to the
preferences of the reader or how they identify, and hopes to be inclusive
and useful to all. Where it refers to affairs of the heart, or the bedroom, feel
free to read 'she' for 'he' and 'bride' for 'groom' or vice versa. As for gender
stereotypes, this has been written for men, because they are so often sent
out into the world without much advice on how to manage in it. That isn't,
however, to suggest men are uniquely useless, that all the problems and
challenges of the world can be reduced to chromosomes, or that women
might not find something useful here. It is big enough to be a sufficiently
hefty projectile, for a start.

Specially commissioned photographs taken by Alastair Jennings, with thanks
to model Oliver Smith, and Brian and Eileen Miller at Frederick L Mabb, Yeovil
(www.frederickmabb.co.uk) for their patience, help and advice.

Photographs supplied by the publishers or Shutterstock, and by Getty on
pages 4, 6, 20, 54, 58, 59 (all), 60 (all), 71 (all), 78, 85 (all), 94, 96, 120 and 142.

CONTENTS

 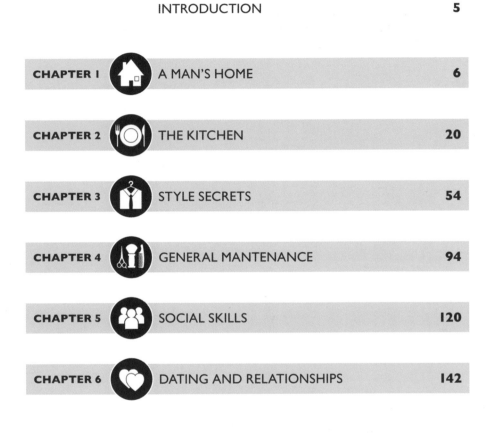

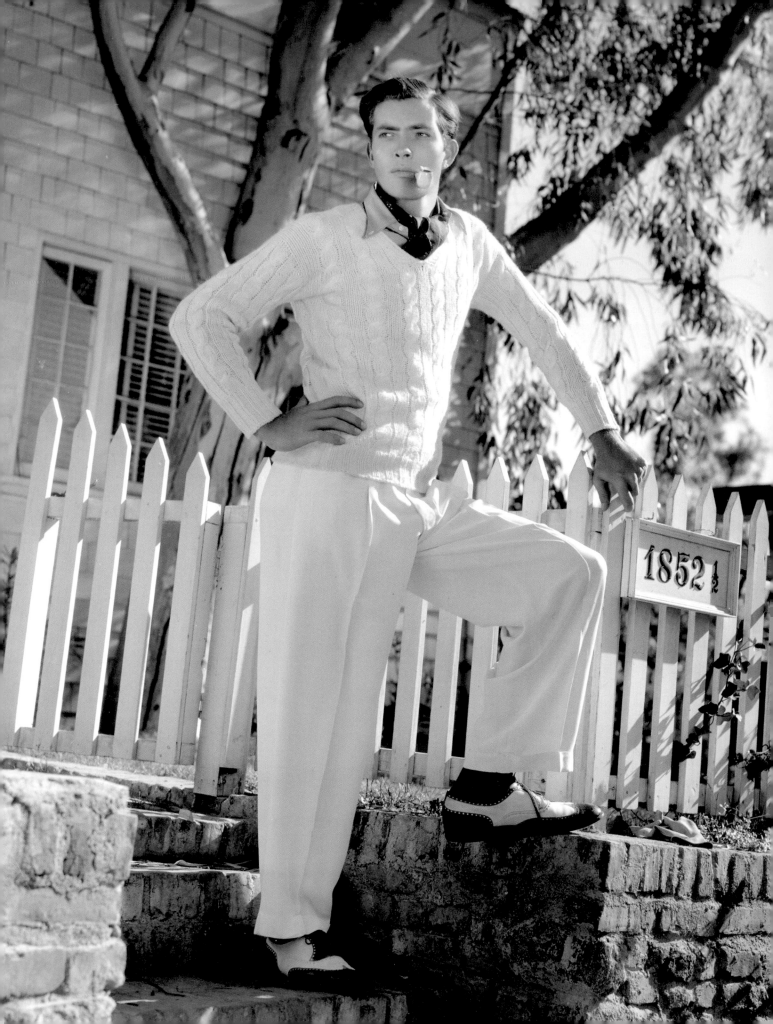

INTRODUCTION

Men, like cars, need looking after. It's perfectly possible to run them on cheap fuel, drive them fast and recklessly, or forget to wash them – they'll still get you from A to B, but the ride won't be smooth, and at some point in the future they will conk out by the side of the road. To perform at their best they require care, regular maintenance and an occasional polish. But cars come with instructions, and men do not. To be allowed to operate a moving vehicle, you have to go through intensive training and pass hard physical and mental tests. All you need to qualify as a man are testicles and an 18th birthday.

We are sent out into the world with very little information on how to navigate it. How to run the body we've got, and manage the demands of the modern world with style. When it is appropriate to move in for a man hug and when to hang back for a handshake. How to talk to total strangers and extricate ourselves gracefully from awkward situations. How to shift a stubborn stain, tie a bow-tie, keep a clean house, shave without cutting ourselves to ribbons. When to tweet and when to put away the phone. How to deliver a killer best-man speech, survive a stag night, dance like you know what you're doing. How to be a man, but more than that – how to be the best man possible.

That's what this book is for. The pages that follow offer advice and guidance on making the best of what you have and steering a stylish path through some of the obstacles life puts in the way. We've included tips on dealing with everyday hassles and pointers on those once-in-a-lifetime pickles in which men can find themselves.

Like all advice, it is best taken with a pinch of salt. Part of the point of youth is to challenge the wisdom of old men, find your own way and make your own mistakes. Centuries of men have learned from the experiences of their fathers and done things better than before, which is why wooden teeth and outside toilets have gone out of style and you are no longer expected to marry your cousin.

Many men are very far from helpless. Some have been raised to cook and clean and trim their nose hair and hold the door open, tie a Windsor knot and make a mean Martini. If you are one of those Renaissance men, and know better than this book on any subject, by all means go with your gut and ignore our suggestions. However, those fully rounded men who scoff at advice would do well to note that one mark of a man is the ability to accept that he can never know it all. There is advice here on the basics, including loading a dishwasher and chopping an onion, because plenty of guys leave home without knowing this stuff, and wind up coming up with their own solutions. Which are random, and only sometimes right.

Your first job here on Earth is to look after yourself. You are the best person for this job because a) you're deeply invested in the outcome, b) you know what makes you tick and c) no one else can be arsed.

For the young man out in the world on his own, looking after himself can feel like a daunting, lonely, thankless prospect. Take heart in the fact that for every problem you encounter, a man (or woman) has met it before and come up with a solution. The best of those are compiled here, to help you become the best man you can be. Enjoy the ride.

Richard Hutt, 2017

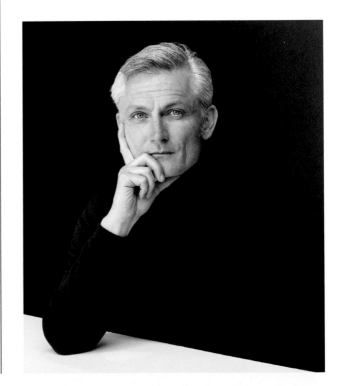

'Style is knowing who you are, what you want to say, and not giving a damn'
Orson Welles

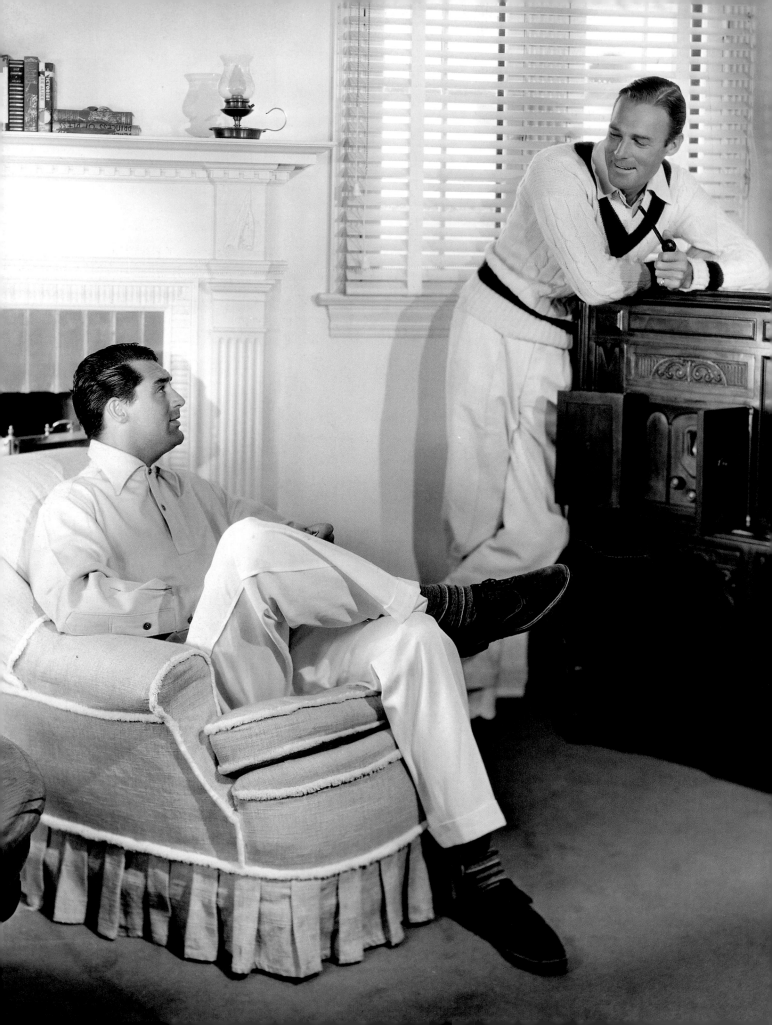

CHAPTER I

A MAN'S HOME

A man's home should be his castle, whether it is a tiny windowless cupboard laughably advertised as a double room, or a glittering penthouse bachelor pad. Whatever the space you inhabit, take the time to seize control of it. With a little effort and the advice that follows, you can be lord of your domain, however pokey.

MAKE YOURSELF AT HOME

The prime difference between a boy and a man is independence. A boy waits for others to look after him; a man does it himself. Self-reliance starts at home. The moment you cross the threshold into manhood, it becomes time for you to learn to do the things that have always been done for you: the cleaning; the cooking; the mystical process that turns dirty pants into clean ones.

Running your own ship

For those just moving out from the family nest and into the world of adult responsibility, there is good news and bad. The good news first – you are free. You can now do pretty much what you want, when you want. As those who moved out a while ago already know, this is also the bad news. You, my son, are on your own. No one is going to lift a finger to help you, unless you pay them to do it, or you debase yourself by taking laundry to your mum (don't). But don't despair. You've got this. There are several reasons to take on the tidying, cleaning, maintaining your own home:

◆ The state of the place in which you live is a reflection of you. Untidy, dirty, dishevelled is not a good look.

◆ If you are single, there is always a possibility a love interest might see where you live. Look around you – would they be turned on or appalled?

◆ It is much, much less depressing to indulge bad habits, such as daytime TV or video games, in a clean and well-organised home. You will feel better about yourself, and spend less time looking for lost keys/wallet/phone.

◆ It's cheaper to clean/maintain things yourself than pay someone else to fix them – which is what will happen if you don't clean and maintain them.

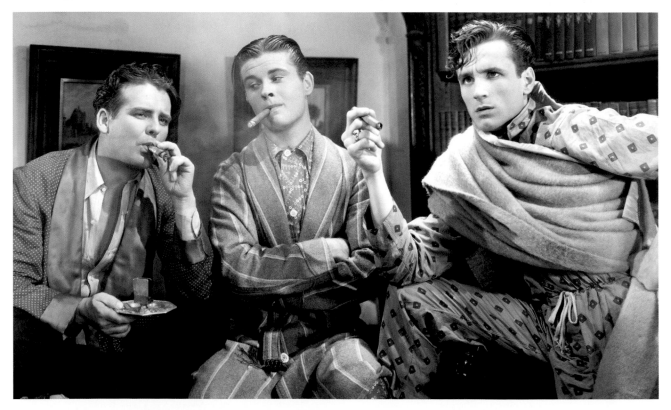

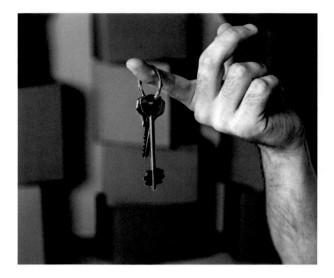

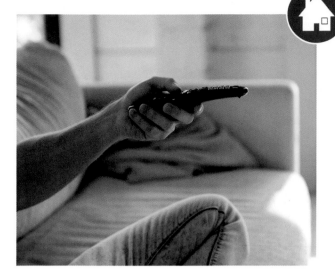

◆ Men who can take care of themselves are less likely to try to find a partner based on their ability to wash their socks/feed them chips. Better reasons for a relationship include attraction, love, affection and mutual interests.

The same principles apply, whether you are living on your own in a bedsit or penthouse, in student halls, a house-share or still at home. Independence rules – look after yourself.

Before you go

If you are about to move out of the family home, think carefully and be honest – can you afford it? Real life contains all kinds of hidden expenses, including a daunting chunk of upfront cash for rent etc. Draw up a truthful budget before you commit, or use an online budgeting tool to help you work out what you can afford.

Once you know what the plan is, draw up a list of what you'll need, based on what isn't provided. At the minimum that is likely to include bedding, towels and kitchen stuff. If you are looking to rent, be ready to move quickly – you're likely to need ID, references, proof of income/employment and of course a pile of money. A credit check is usual, and you may need a guarantor.

Sharing a space

For most people, their first living experience outside the family home will involve cohabiting, something that requires patience, sensitivity and a special set of skills. Whether you are sharing a space with fellow students, a partner or flatmates, self-sufficiency is the name of the game. Take responsibility for your actions. In every household there will always be one nightmare – the person who finishes the milk and doesn't replace it, or leaves a dirty ring around the bath and congealed porridge in the sink. Your goal as a flatmate is simple: don't be the asshole. For an easy life, free of drama, learn to share the space considerately.

Making it personal

It's a tough world out there, and a man needs a refuge, a place in which he can be himself and relax. Some men find it easy to live with whatever was there when they moved in, getting by with furniture that just about does the job. It doesn't have to be that way. True, there are limits to what can be done on a budget or in a shared place, but a moderate amount of effort and creativity can create a stylish pad and a welcoming sanctuary from very little indeed.

Deciding on your style

Everyone's idea of luxury is different. If yours is an expensive corporate hotel room, by all means try and recreate it at home. If you've got money to spend, focus on aspects of the room that are most important to your lifestyle and habits and drop the cash there. So, if you spend 12 hours a day in bed, treat yourself to a great mattress. If A/V and gaming are your great pleasures, invest in an oversized TV – or even

Rules for cohabiting

◆ Carve out a space that's yours alone – usually the bedroom. Make this your comfort zone. Pimp it out and be ready to retreat there.
◆ Eat only what's yours.
◆ Clean up after yourself.
◆ For communal stuff, use a kitty – everyone contributes money to the pot, which is used for toilet paper, milk, etc.
◆ For chores everyone hates, use a rota.
◆ Whatever is bothering you, let it go. People are weird, including you. If the habits of your flatmates are so annoying you can't be in the same room as them, leave the room.

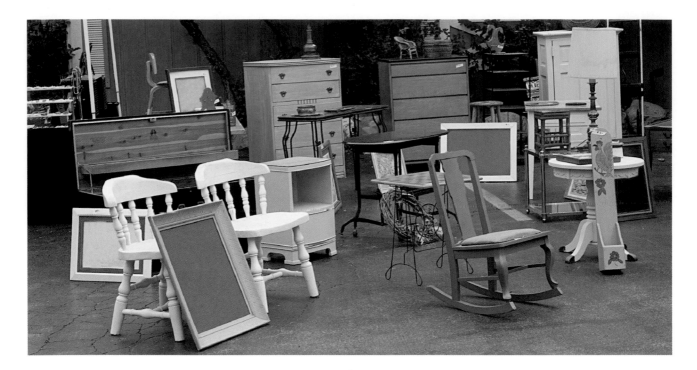

a projector, screen and blackout blinds (NB: an unsightly sprawl of cables ruins the sleek look – hide/tidy them).

If you want a timeless bachelor-pad look, and can afford the hefty price tag, buy design classics. Mid-century chairs by Eames, Bertoia, Saarinen, etc hold their value well and are as pleasing to use as they are to look at. Or save your money and buy reproductions – non-licensed versions of old-school armchairs are readily available.

If your budget is somewhat more shoestring, don't despair. The odds are that almost anything you could buy from Ikea was bought, not that long ago, by someone who lives near you and who now wants rid of it. Try junk yards, eBay, charity/thrift stores, flea markets, car boot sales. Old stuff is generally cooler than new stuff and for the most part the only 'upcycling' you'll have to do is cleaning.

Decor

If you aren't renting – or if you are, and the landlord is cool with you making improvements – a pot of paint and a weekend can transform the space. Take the time to get it right; 70% of a good paint job is prep work, particularly masking off the areas you don't want painted, to get clean edges. White is always OK, particularly if you've got colour elsewhere, but don't be suckered into thinking it's the only option. Dark colours can work surprisingly well in the most windowless room, as can a feature wall picked out in one vivid colour. If you've got a lot of ground to cover and trustworthy friends, organise a painting party, with payment in pizza or similar.

Frames are cheap. So are reproductions of classic film posters, prints of photos you love, LP covers, etc.

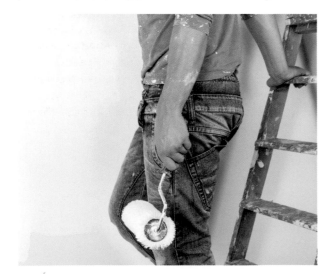

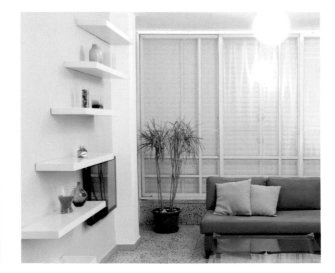

Choose images carefully, mirroring colours in the room and reflecting you and your tastes – and that you are happy to look at endlessly. If you have money to spend, invest in art (or vintage posters) that means something to you, and use a professional framer to make it look good. Mirrors add light, make the space appear bigger, and allow you to check yourself from multiple angles. Not over the bed please.

Instead of a blinding central light that washes out the space, buy lamps (second-hand ones are fine) and use them to mark out zones via the light they cast. So, get a reading lamp for the armchair you like to sit in, a standard (tall) lamp for the TV corner, a bedside light for bed-based activities. The variety of options gives you control over the mood, and lifts the vibe and the spirit instantly.

After lamps, the quickest, cheapest way to pimp the space is a rug. For old-school masculine luxury and underfoot comfort, it's hard to beat sheepskin – otherwise, aim for colours reflecting any soft furnishings. A throw may not be the first thing a man envisages when he thinks of a bachelor pad, but a well-chosen fabric draped over the bed or sofa can help soften a stark space and make minimal feel luxurious. Ditto cushions, which are cheap and add comfort. Think about texture as well as colour.

Organising your space

Draw a plan of your living space and sketch in any existing furniture. Think about what you like to do, and how rearranging things into dedicated zones might make it easier. So, if you like to watch TV in bed, or need a space in which to read, set up the room around those interests. Some items are non-negotiable (you will always want your sofa to be the right distance from the TV), which helps narrow down your options. Draw lines to indicate the way you would usually walk around the space and ensure these pathways are clear.

▾ With furnishing, less is often more. Minimalism demands tidiness.

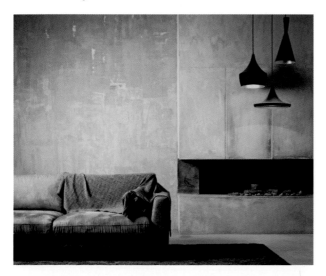

Home cleaning routine

Life is hard and stuff doesn't clean itself. Happily, I promise you have the requisite skills. And doing it will remind you of that, and your independence. It'll also mean you have a healthier, happier space in which to live, which you won't be ashamed to let someone else see.

Set yourself a routine. Don't let stuff pile up, figuratively or literally. The following is a rough guide – make your own, based on the time available and your priorities.

◆ On a daily basis you need to: make the bed; wash the dishes; clean kitchen surfaces (wipe with a sponge and spray cleaner); sweep the kitchen floor; put dirty clothes in the laundry; and spray and wipe the shower after use.
◆ Once a week, at the very least, you need to: clean toilets, the shower, bathroom sinks, the bath and mirrors; hoover carpets; mop hard floors; and give everything a good old dust.
◆ About once a month – or every few months depending on how often you cook and where you live (cities are grimier places than the countryside) – you need to: clean the oven (use a spray-on/walk-away cleaner); clean the windows.

Stuff and how to store it

The best way to manage stuff is to own nothing. Assuming you are not Gandhi, that may feel a bit extreme, and possessions are comforting things to have around. To maximise impact, be as ruthless as you can when assessing what can be got rid of (keeping only what you truly love or need) and as organised as possible when working out where what remains should go. Create a rule and a home for every item. And then (this is the hard part) put it there. Always. If you live alone and leave your pants on the floor, you will return to find your pants still on the floor. You are a man, and this is no way to live. Buy a laundry basket.

Yes, they are for reading, but books also display worldly wisdom and wide-ranging tastes in an effective visual shorthand that is pleasing on the eye. Ditto records, vintage video-game cartridges, snow globes, whatever. In an increasingly digital world, retro analogue possessions add charm and character. If, like many men, you have a collection of stuff, work out how best to display it.

HOW TO
KEEP IT CLEAN

Washing up

We're starting with the worst job, which is a good strategy for life and for facing a kitchen nightmare. If you don't have a dishwasher you'll want to optimise your approach. Equip yourself properly: sponge with scouring pad; brush; washing-up bowl; washing-up liquid; washing-up gloves; dish rack. Follow a system and it will be done before you know it.

1 Stack everything dirty to one side of the sink, by type – glasses, plates, cutlery, pans – scraping food residue into the bin.
2 Pans with stuck-on stuff need soaking – fill with cold water and leave to one side overnight.
3 Fill the sink or washing-up bowl with the hottest water your hands can cope with and a squeeze of liquid. Plates with stuff crusted to them can be left to soak at the bottom of the sink/bowl. The same does *not* apply to knives!
4 Scrub each item until it's clean, fiddly stuff first, then cutlery – it really needs to be clean.
5 After scrubbing, rinse with hot water. Use a separate washing-up bowl if you have one – rinsing them under the tap works but wastes water.
6 Stack washed items in the rack to air dry, or use a *clean* tea towel to dry them.
7 Do those pans you soaked and were thinking about ignoring. Use a brush, especially if cleaning a non-stick pan. For burnt-on foods, fill the pan with water, put it on the hob and heat until it's boiling. Turn off the heat and use a spatula or similar to scrape off the burnt bits before washing it.

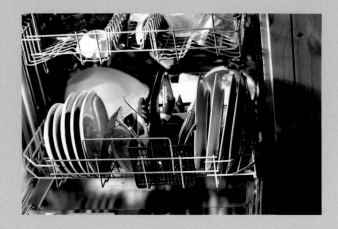

Using a dishwasher

If you have one, make the most of it. Loading and unloading a dishwasher is a pain in the ass, but it is less of a pain than washing up – so suck it up and be grateful.

1 Make sure you've removed all food residues.
2 If plates etc are going to sit there all day, rinse them before loading.
3 There's a dedicated space for everything, use it. Stacking bowls on top of bowls will mean they don't get washed.
4 Don't jam the machine with stuff – it won't work as well.
5 Clean the filter regularly and, once in a while, give the machine a deep clean.

Laundry

This is where most male at-home mishaps occur. Take care, or your whites will be pink, your blacks grey, and your jumpers laughably small. Separate the clothes into piles: whites, darks, colours, and sensitive things you can't put

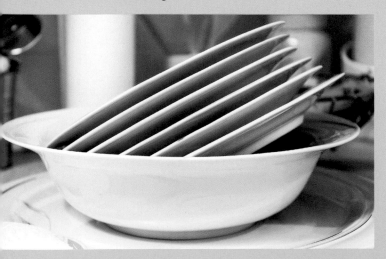

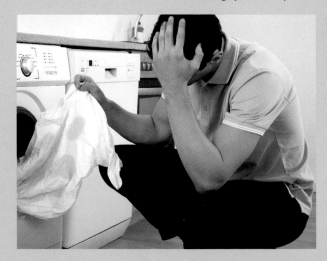

in a washing machine. Whites are any light clothes, from white to light blue. Sensitive stuff includes wool and silk. READ THE LABEL. PS Empty pockets!

Fill the washing machine. DON'T OVERFILL or it won't wash properly. Choose the setting appropriate for the colour and dirt factor. White cotton shirts can be washed fairly hot (40°C/100°F) but be aware that the hotter you go the shorter the life of the shirt. If in doubt, go colder – 30°C/86°F is a good compromise. Towels and (white) sheets like it hot – 60°C/140°F is fine.

Add detergent. Turn on. Wait. When the wash cycle is finished, take out the clothes, shake and hang to dry promptly; damp clothes smell and wrinkle. Tumble-drying is fine, though hard on clothes but the best option is outside – they'll smell nicer, it doesn't waste electricity, and it costs nothing. If drying inside, hang them on a clothes rack somewhere warm with decent ventilation.

Bedding

I've known men who only changed their sheets when they thought someone else might see them – if what someone else thinks is more important than how you feel, have a word with yourself. Polls show that on average men don't believe bedding becomes disgusting enough to warrant a change until about six weeks in. You spend one-third of your life in bed – why would you settle for a crumpled, smelly environment when crisp, fragrant, clean is so easily achieved? If you want to feel clean and sleep well, change your sheets once a week. If you can't cope with that, give yourself two weeks.

Cotton sheets are a safe bet – buy the best you can afford (this is advice we are going to be repeating). A good rule of thumb is thread count. Anything above 200 is likely to be decent quality, feel good and last. Poly-cotton blends are cheaper and dry quickly, but can have an artificial feel. Buy fitted sheets – elasticated at the sides and shaped to the mattress – or learn to make hospital corners.

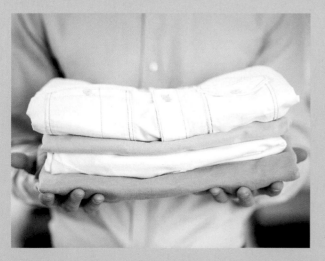

Clothes labels

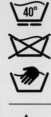 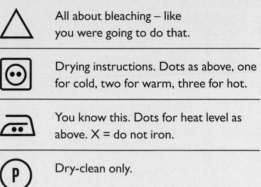

40°	If it has a number in it, that's the max/right temperature. If dots, then one for cold, two for warm, three for hot. X in a bucket = don't wash, dry-clean only. Picture of a hand means wash by hand only.
△	All about bleaching – like you were going to do that.
⊡	Drying instructions. Dots as above, one for cold, two for warm, three for hot.
🔲	You know this. Dots for heat level as above. X = do not iron.
Ⓟ	Dry-clean only.

Removing stains

Grass: Soak clothes in cold water, apply detergent directly to the stain, rub it in, wash as normal.

Mud: Wait until the mud is dry, brush it off, apply detergent, wash as normal.

Ink: Treat as quickly as possible. If you can't deal with it immediately, at least soak up the ink with a cloth. Don't scrub, just blot. Apply a water-based cleaning agent ASAP and blot again. If it worked, wash as normal – but don't put anything else in the machine at the same time.

Wine: Blot it, soaking up as much liquid as you can. Hold the marked area over an empty bowl and sprinkle salt generously on the stain. Then pour over very hot water, keeping the fabric taut. Wash as normal.

Gum: Put the item in the freezer, then chip off the gum and wash as normal.

HOME MAINTENANCE

The transition to manhood is about learning to do for yourself what others once did for you. Your home, and the things in it, are now your responsibility (and your landlord's, if you are renting). Taking the time to deal with essential tasks, to own the space and make it yours, will give you a sense of independence – calling your dad for help changing a light bulb will not.

Know your home

Before you start (ideally, when you move in) familiarise yourself with the locations of a few key devices. Trying to fix a leaking tap without knowing how to turn off the water supply is a stupid idea, liable to flood your kitchen – as 'someone I know' once found out, to his wife's great annoyance. You should, at least, be able to locate your electricity meter, fuse box/consumer box, gas meter, gas mains tap, water meter and stopcock, allowing you to monitor and turn off the water/gas/electricity coming into

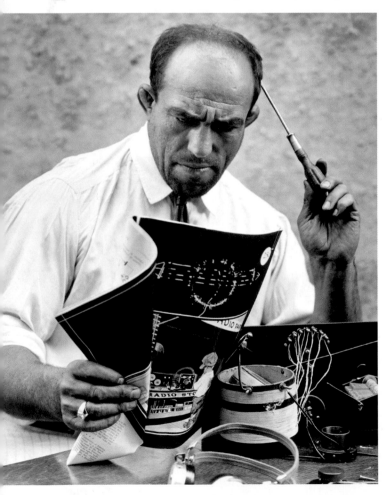

the home and thus limit the amount of damage/death you can bring into your space. Hopefully.

If you live in a rented place, the landlord will be responsible for most repairs, including anything to do with the structure/exterior; plumbing; heating/hot water; gas appliances and electrical wiring. Before making repairs yourself, check the tenancy agreement – you may not be permitted to do much, in case you make a mess of it or yourself. Legally, you can't be forced to make repairs that are the landlord's responsibility.

Basic maintenance tasks

You don't have to be an expert plumber, electrician or handyman to master a few basic tasks. Learning to change a fuse and bleed a radiator will give you confidence in your ability to look after things for yourself. Once you've got the little things down you can build your skills and take on the more challenging projects.

The tool rule

Nothing will make you feel more of a man than your own toolbox, even if it only contains a torch and a pocket screwdriver. The tool rule is consistent with all the other advice in this book: buy the best you can afford. You want this stuff to hang around for years. See what you can scavenge off parents and other family members before investing heavily in diamond-tipped power tools. Big, expensive bits of kit likely to be used infrequently (such as floor-sanders) can be rented when needed.

Health and safety

Know your limits – if a DIY task involves things that can cause serious bodily harm, leave it to the professionals and GSI (Get Someone In). Accident and Emergency departments are full of men who thought they knew how to operate a power saw.

TOOLS OF THE TRADE

Multi-tool

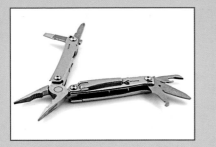

This is cheating, but if you can afford only one object, a good multi-tool is a great place to start. It incorporates pliers, screwdrivers, etc in one handy package.

Screwdrivers

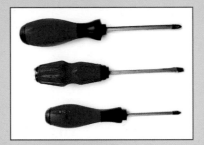

You'll need a range of sizes, in flat and Phillips (star-shape) heads, and they should be comfortable to grip so try before you buy. Magnetic tips make things easier.

Hammer

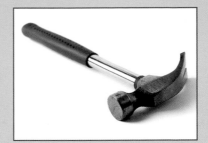

Is there a manlier object than a hammer? No. A claw-head one will allow you to extract the nails you have enthusiastically banged into the wrong places.

Tape measure

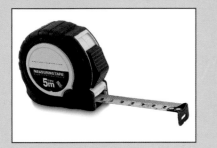

Nothing makes a DIY project fail quicker than guesswork. Buy a tape measure, and use it carefully. 'Measure twice, cut once' said a very wise man.

Spirit level

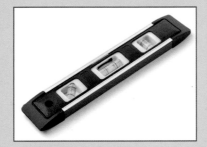

There's an app for ensuring your hung items are straight, but using it isn't as satisfying as establishing a straight line by means of a stick with a little bubble in it.

Wrench

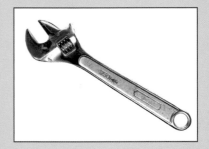

Buy an adjustable wrench and you will have no need of a range of spanners. It's good for tightening and loosening anything that moves — nuts and plumbing fittings in particular.

Drill

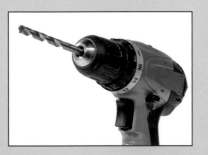

Cordless ones are handy and portable, but electric drills are powerful and versatile. Using a good drill correctly delivers intense man-satisfaction levels.

Saw

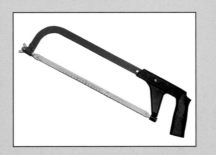

A hacksaw with replaceable blades should do you for most household tasks, such as the removal of stray bits of wood, plastic pipe, etc.

Allen/hex keys

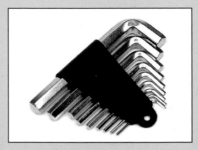

These hexagonal little keys will unlock a world of flat-pack wonder. They are often supplied along with the million screws and incomprehensible instructions, so just hang on to them as you go.

HOW TO
CHANGE A LIGHT BULB

Yes, this is easy, but that doesn't mean it is impossible to get wrong.

Equipment
New light bulb.

1 Choose the same wattage bulb as the one you had in there before, assuming it didn't give you problems. Make sure you choose the correct fitting – bayonet is the one with the two prong bits, screw looks like … a screw.

2 The first needs a gentle push in before you turn it anticlockwise to remove it. Turn off the light before replacing the bulb, or risk a rude shock. If the bulb was on recently, let it cool before touching it.

3 For high ceilings, use an actual ladder or step stool, with someone holding it, rather than a random stack of furniture.

4 A broken light bulb can be removed with needle-nose pliers and a lot of care – turn off the power at the breaker first.

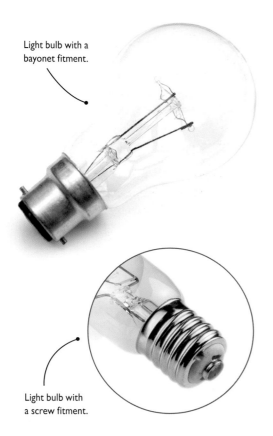

Light bulb with a bayonet fitment.

Light bulb with a screw fitment.

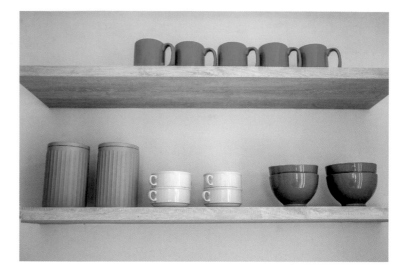

HOW TO
PUT UP A FLOATING SHELF

What you can hang, where, depends on the wall and what's behind it. If it's sturdy solid brick or masonry then life is relatively simple. If it is plasterboard, start by locating the studs – the wooden uprights to which the plasterboard is affixed. Knock on the wall until you find a spot that doesn't sound hollow – or buy a stud detector, which will also let you know if you are about to drill into pipes or cables. If you are fixing the shelf to a solid wall, you don't need to find the studs, but be sure to use a masonry drill bit and solid wall plugs.

Equipment
Measuring tape, spirit level, stud detector, drill, wall plugs, screws, brackets, shelf.

1 Once you've checked for pipes and cables, mark holes for the first bracket by holding it in place, sticking a pencil into the fixing holes and drawing a little cross in the centre of each (if the bracket is too thick for the pencil, use a wire to make the mark).

2 Choose the right size drill bit for the plugs, and plugs the right size for the screws, then drill the hole and fix the first bracket into position. Don't over-tighten the screws.

3 Place the shelf into position on the bracket and insert the other bracket.

4 Using your spirit level – and another pair of hands, if available – mark the position of the new bracket.

5 Drill and fix as above, and again, don't tighten up until you've checked it is straight.

NB Do not attempt to fix a very heavy item to plasterboard only – though there are wall plugs designed to help you do this, it is possible that one sunny day it will come down … bringing a chunk of wall with it.

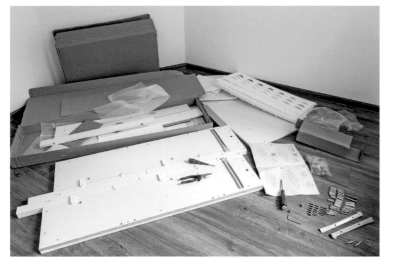

HOW TO
ASSEMBLE FLAT-PACK FURNITURE

The reason large Swedish furniture shops can sell sofas cheaply is because you and I are prepared to do the work – an arrangement that has caused many men to weep hot tears of regret. With the right approach, however, this can be significantly less painful. Dress comfortably, have the correct tools to hand and an assistant within shouting distance. Put on some music. This will take a while.

Equipment
Allen/hex key (usually provided), power or manual screwdriver, patience.

1 Work in the room the item is going in. The significance of this advice will become clear the moment you finish assembling a wardrobe that won't fit through the door.

2 Unpack everything and lay it out. Working on the flattened cardboard, laid on the floor, helps protect the furniture and carpet.

3 Check the parts list. If there is a fixing missing, replace it before you go any further. The allen/hex key should be included (if not, now's the time to draw on your accumulated cache in your toolbox). Check the major parts aren't damaged.

4 You can use a power screwdriver to help you assemble the item, but only with care – it's easy to over-tighten and put a hole in the cheap chipboard, so it's better to finish the job by hand. Put all the fiddly bits to one side.

5 Sit down and read the instructions through to the end. It doesn't matter if you don't understand why they have done things in a certain order – follow the instructions and use the right piece in the right place.

6 If you despair or hit a wall, work backwards through the instructions to find any errors you may have made, or Google it to find out how others coped.

HOW TO
CHANGE A FUSE

A fuse is a small device designed to stop the electric current when there is a fault. For appliances, fuses live inside plugs and, for the household, a consumer box – the item formerly known as the fuse box. If an electrical item goes kaput it's possible the fuse needs replacing.

Equipment
Flat-headed screwdriver, replacement fuse.

1 Check whether the plug has a fuse holder. If it does, open it up with the flat-headed screwdriver. If not, undo the large screw in the middle of the plug and open it.

2 Fish out the (cylindrical) fuse and replace it with one that has same amperage as the one you are removing (3A or 13A, depending on the device).

3 If you replace a fuse and the device still doesn't work, there's a problem somewhere else. Call an electrician, or buy a new hairdryer.

Household fuses (circuit breakers) operate in a similar way: they disconnect the electricity supply to a circuit in the home, generally because something has gone wrong, such as someone has overloaded the circuit with electrical items. Given the variety of systems and the high risk factor, we won't attempt to give you instructions, but generally these fuses can be switched out like the fuses in plugs. However, if you feel out of your depth/don't own a multi-meter, leave it to the pros. Electricity can kill.

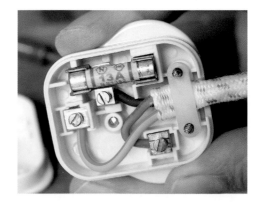

HOW TO
UNBLOCK THE TOILET

We've all done it, though we may not have admitted to it. Whatever is down there, deal with it as soon as you notice and before it starts overflowing on the floor. If it is blocked, don't flush – it will make things worse.

Equipment
Chemical drain unblocker and gloves OR goggles, long rubber gloves, small plunger, strong plastic bag, disinfectant.

1 The nastiness of the matter involved means you may forgive yourself for buying some chemicals and chucking them down the toilet. Again, handle with care.

2 If you are going manual, come equipped – goggles and long rubber gloves and a small plunger, with a strong plastic bag (no holes) for any waste you extract. If you are feeling manful and the gloves are long enough, just close your eyes, insert a hand, and feel for the blockage – you may be able to loosen any wads of toilet paper etc manually.

3 If not, have at it with the plunger. Start gently or risk a nasty clean-up job. Flush to check it has worked.

4 Stick any waste in the bag and take it to an outside bin, then disinfect yourself and anything you used or touched.

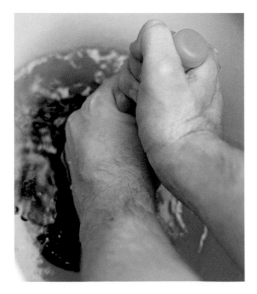

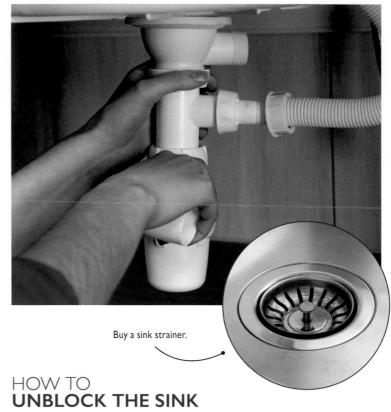

Buy a sink strainer.

HOW TO
UNBLOCK THE SINK

The easiest way to unblock the sink is, of course, to not block it in the first place. Buy a sink strainer. It collects the food bits that would otherwise go down the plughole and block the drains, and is the best money you will spend this year.

Equipment
Chemical sink unblocker and gloves OR cloth, plunger and gloves, AND POSSIBLY washing-up bowl, plumbers snake or auger.

1 Sinks can be unblocked manually or with chemicals. If you're lazy, buy a product and chuck it down there, but follow the instructions exactly, particularly the safety tips – that is some nasty and corrosive stuff.

2 If you prefer not to use gunk, block the overflow with a cloth, fill the sink with water, and position a plunger over the plughole. Then go at it manfully, pumping the handle vigorously to dislodge the offending material.

3 If that didn't work, you may need to get under the sink and look for the blockage. Put a bucket or washing-up bowl under the pipes and unscrew the U-shaped section.

4 Clean out the pipe in another sink. Reassemble with care and check you did so by running the tap and looking for drips with the bucket or bowl still in place.

5 If that still didn't work, resort to the nasty chemical stuff or keep going further down the pipes, using a plumber's snake or auger to dislodge whatever it is. Now buy a sink strainer.

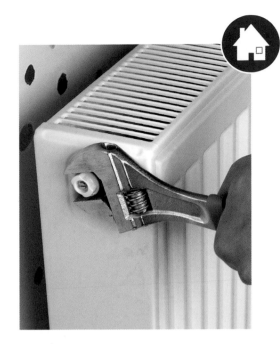

HOW TO
FIX A DRIPPING TAP

Start by turning off the water supply. There's probably an isolation valve under the sink – look for an accessible valve on the pipe with a screw in it. If the line on the screw head is vertical (in line with the pipe) the supply is on – in which case insert a screwdriver and turn it through one-quarter of a revolution so it is horizontal to the pipe. If you can't find one of these, turn off the water at the main stopcock.

Equipment
Wrench, screwdriver.

1 Run the taps to get rid of any water in the system and to check you have indeed turned it off.

2 Put the plug in the sink (this limits the risk of something fiddly getting lost down the plughole).

3 You probably need to replace either a rubber washer or a ceramic disc, depending on the type of tap. Check by turning it – if it will only go a half-turn, it is ceramic, and you'll need to replace the whole valve. With a rubber washer you will only need to replace the ring.

4 Get inside the tap by removing the handle. Find the handle screw – often hidden under a cap on the handle, which can be unscrewed or prised off. Unscrew the handle and you can get at the parts.

5 Keep all the bits you remove somewhere safe, set out in the order in which you took them off.

6 You should now see the valve. If it has a metal cover (shroud), take it off. Loosen the valve with the wrench so you can remove it, while holding the tap with your other hand. The washer is located at the bottom of the valve. Replace it with a new, identical washer. Reassemble.

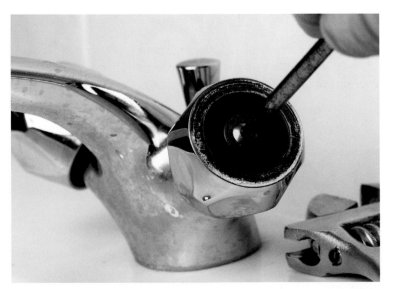

HOW TO
BLEED A RADIATOR

Over time, air bubbles can get trapped in your heating system, meaning it doesn't work as effectively as it could – if your radiators have cold spots, you need to bleed them.

Equipment
Cloths x 2, dish, radiator key.

1 Before you get started, check there isn't anything more serious going on. Make sure the boiler pilot light is on, and look for rust or water underneath or on the radiator – this could indicate there are leaks in the system. Turn off the system before you begin, unless you enjoy being sprayed with boiling water.

2 Insert a radiator key to fit the square bleed screw in the side of the top corner of the radiator. Hold it with a cloth, and put a dish or another cloth under the valve in case of drips. Turn the key slooooowly, anticlockwise. You will hear a hissing sound – be ready with the second cloth.

3 When the sound stops, tighten again. Don't try to prove your strength by over-tightening, which can damage it.

4 Turn on the heating again, and check it's working. Make sure none of the bled radiators are dripping. Job done.

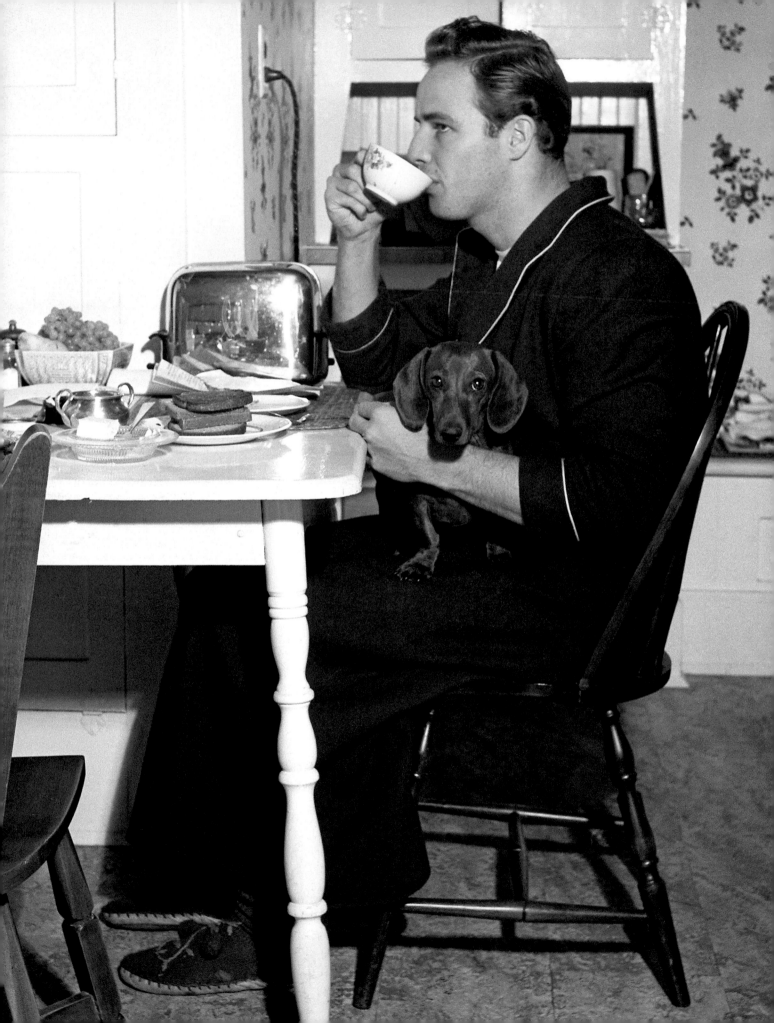

CHAPTER 2

THE KITCHEN

If there is one arena that sorts the men from the boys, it is the kitchen. Cooking is one of the most impressive and useful skills a man can master. It keeps you healthy, makes your life more interesting and saves money. It also demonstrates you have taste, that you can look after yourself and others and aren't so helpless that you have to rely on a parent or a takeaway. Nothing is guaranteed to impress a prospective partner more.

KITCHEN SURVIVAL

A man can run on anything with the basic properties of fuel, and you can survive without knowing how to cook. There are supermarket chains happy to sell you microwaveable plastic tubs of plastic goo containing five days' worth of your recommended saturated fats. And there are always chips. And pizza. And kebabs. You won't thrive on this diet, but you won't die. Not immediately.

However, if you want more than just survival – a long and healthy life; a sense of well-being; the ability to fit into narrow jeans – then you will need to make some effort. Learning to make yourself tasty, nutritious meals you enjoy is liberating and empowering. Because ultimately, no one cares what you eat. Apart from maybe your mum, but this is not her job anymore.

Store-cupboard classics

Doing a 'big shop' and stocking your cupboards with essentials will ensure you are always ready – for uninvited guests, moments when there is nothing edible in the fridge, zombie attack. Well-chosen store-cupboard basics will form the core of your everyday diet, supplemented by fresh veg, fruit, dairy and proteins. We've listed here some classics to stock up on.

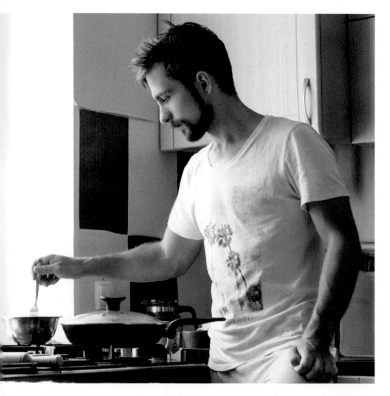

- Pasta – buy the good Italian stuff; extruded through bronze for a rougher texture, it holds the sauce well.
- Noodles – with a packet of noodles (egg, rice, udon, soba) and some soy sauce you are already halfway to dinner. NB flavoured instant noodle packets are jam-packed full of salt and MSG. Make your own.
- Rice – brown is good for you but can be tiresome to cook and eat. Basmati is good quality, and you'll need arborio or carnaroli for risotto. Apart from when making risotto, always rinse rice until the water runs clear, or give it a good long soak.
- Couscous – easy, quick, tasty, this is a store-cupboard lifesaver. Pair it with roast veg and feta cheese for a simple dinner.
- Oats – get in the habit of making porridge, muesli or granola (see 'Quick breakfasts' on p34).
- Canned goods – tomatoes (it's worth buying good-quality ones, since they are less watery); tuna/salmon/anchovies/sardines; chickpeas; beans (can be bought cheaper dried, but most need overnight soaking. Cannellini or butter/lima beans are great for adding to pasta, while pinto or kidney beans are best for chilli since they have a more robust flavour and texture).
- Passata – this is essentially bottled strained tomatoes, and is thicker and smoother than chopped canned tomatoes.
- Tomato paste – this intense red gloop packs a mighty tomato punch, without all the liquid of passata or canned tomatoes.
- Sugar – brown, white (caster/superfine is the most versatile type).
- Salt and pepper – fine table salt is useful (and cheap) for everyday seasoning while cooking, but it is also worth having sea salt flakes and a grinder for seasoning at the table, alongside peppercorns and a grinder.
- Oils – a good olive oil for salads and a cheaper oil for cooking. Sunflower or rapeseed is good for frying etc and sesame adds flavour to a stir-fry.
- Vinegars – wine vinegars (red and white) and balsamic for dressings.

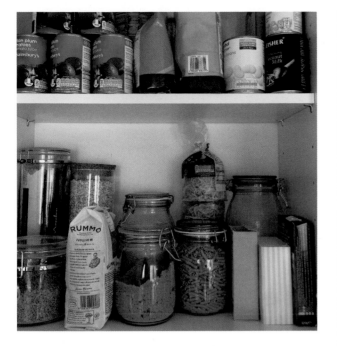

- Capers and canned anchovies – the piquant berries can be used in place of salt as a seasoning in slow-cooked dishes, in which they melt, or whole to lift a salad or add interest to a pizza or bowl of pasta (garlic, lemon zest, capers and chilli and you are there). Ditto anchovies, which are feisty little fish that come in small cans. You only need a couple of fillets, and don't use any additional salt.
- Flour – plain/all-purpose and self-raising. You need this for coating and thickening as well as baking. Cornflour/corn starch is really useful for making sauces since it doesn't leave behind a raw flour taste and is less likely to produce lumps. Baking powder is required in many baking recipes.
- Stock – good-quality instant granules are readily available. Look for those without MSG.
- Herbs – for a slow-cooked recipe, use dried herbs, for adding at the end use fresh. Buy a growing plant, keeping it alive on the windowsill as long as possible with water and light. Parsley, basil, thyme, mint, rosemary – all can elevate almost any dish.
- Spices – go to town on spices – the cheapest way to bring flavour and variety to the plate. Buying new spices as you try out recipes will help you build up a comprehensive backlist of tastes – sealed, they keep well. Standards include peppercorns, paprika, curry powder, garam masala, bay leaves, dried chilli, fennel seeds, nutmeg, cinnamon, star anise.
- Long-life essentials – there are a few essentials it is worth always keeping in the fridge: lemons; garlic; ginger; onions (and shallots if you want to be fancy); eggs (free-range); frozen peas; Parmesan cheese.

Condiments of the gods

It is likely that a lot of your fridge space will be taken up by sauces, because a man knows that nothing is more dispiriting than the prospect of a fried-egg sandwich without ketchup.

- Worcester Sauce – jazzes up cheese on toast, goes brilliantly with mushrooms, adds zing to steak and Bolognese sauce.
- Sriracha – this spicy and flavourful red sauce is good with eggs or any rice dish.
- Fish sauce – a powerful liquid made from fermented fish, this adds punch, salt and umami to fish dishes and curries.
- Ketchup – there are lots of types out there, some of which are sinfully sweet and salty, while others pack a more tomatoey, less synthetic punch. Take your pick.
- Mayonnaise – having a jar of this creamy goo to hand means even the blandest sandwich or salad can be made more luxurious.
- Mustard – at the very least you'll need Dijon for salad dressings/sandwiches and English for smearing on your sausages.
- Mango chutney – great with cheese, exceptional with or in curry – stir a generous spoonful in at the end to bring sweetness and tang.
- Balsamic vinegar – ideal for salad dressings, but also desserts, drizzles, glazes, and thrown liberally into tomato sauces.
- Tamari soy sauce – a dark, rich Japanese soy sauce, this is generally less salty than its Chinese cousin. It ramps up Asian cooking – noodles are nothing without it – but keep an eye on your sodium levels.
- Harissa – this North African spice paste is hot, rich and flavourful – great with couscous, tagines, chicken, etc.

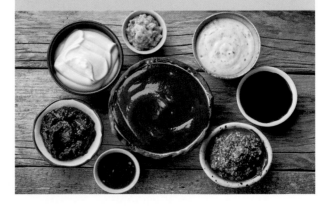

KITCHEN EQUIPMENT

You can achieve a lot with a knife, a pan, and a wooden spoon, but to run your kitchen with minimum hassle, it's worth investing in a bit of kit. Before you go crazy, be sure to check what you can scrounge off family and friends – people are always getting rid of kitchen stuff to make room for more kitchen stuff. Here's a list of the most useful basics:

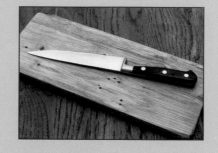

Chef's knife
The chef's knife is the one knife to rule them all – a classic, versatile object that can cope with chopping, slicing, mincing and more.

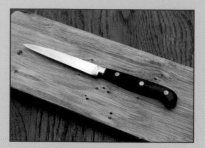

Paring knife
Ideal for most fiddly smaller jobs. A serrated bread knife is also useful. Avoid buying knife sets, which tend to be a false economy since many include knives you will never need.

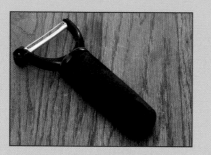

Y-shaped peeler
Having a peeler saves time, food and fingers. NB peelings can be useful – see 'Love your leftovers' on p33.

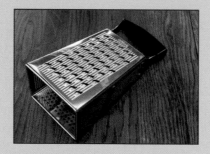

Graters of varying sizes
Or a box-style one that has several sides to it. For lemons, ginger, etc, an ultra-sharp Microplane-style grater is a good investment – just mind your fingers.

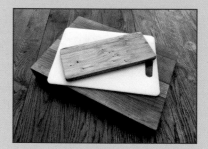

Several chopping boards
Heavy plastic is easier to deal with than wood and can go in the dishwasher, where it will be properly disinfected.

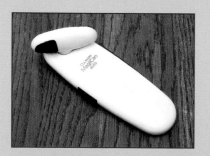

Can opener
If you want to annoy yourself forever, buy a cheap one.

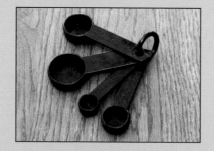

Measuring jugs/spoons
Most recipes should be followed carefully until you have nailed them. Baking in particular needs the precision you get with proper measuring spoons/jug.

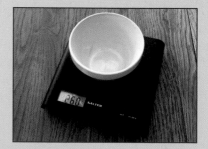

Scales
Digital ones are cheap, accurate, and take up little space.

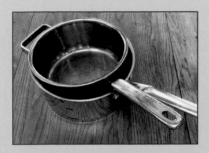

A set of heavy pans
As a rule of thumb, the heavier the pan, the better it is to cook with. Avoid plastic handles – you may want to put them in the oven, or under the grill/broiler.

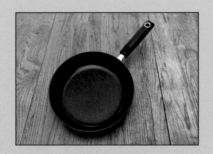

Frying pans
One large and one small. Non-stick is good since it means you can use less fat, but take care of it – no metal spatulas or abrasive scouring pads.

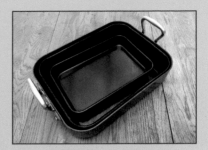

Roasting pans
Again, go for heavy ones if possible. Essential for a proper roast, and saving the precious juices from meat for gravy etc. Buy non-stick, or rue the day you didn't.

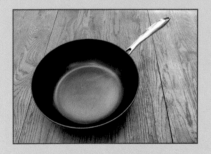

Wok
Stir-frying is hard work unless you have a good wok. Buy something big enough to cook for more than one, and look after it – oil regularly to avoid rust.

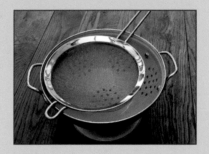

Colander and sieve
Unexciting but vital, the colander will drain your noodles/pasta/spuds, the sieve is for rinsing your veg/herbs/rice.

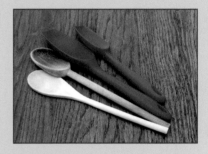

Spoons
A home cook can get quite attached to a wooden spoon – use for stirring, tasting. Silicone spoons and spatulas are dishwasher safe.

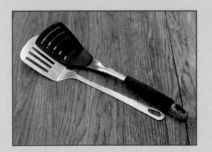

Fish slice
For flipping stuff in the pan (fish fillets, burgers, eggs, etc) or scraping the good bits out of it.

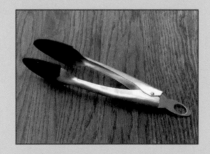

Tongs
For precision control in a pan/meat/fish scenario, and for removing things safely from boiling water, where you really don't want an improvised solution.

Other items
- Kitchen scissors
- Bottle opener/corkscrew
- Plates, bowls, glasses, cutlery, mugs. Buy a set if you can – or again, scrounge. Lots of mismatched plates can actually be a good look.
- Blender – a 'stick' blender is cheap, and is the one plug-in kitchen device that is most likely to actually get used, for blitzing sauces and soups in seconds.

How to shop

Supermarket shopping is a war, and you are in the middle of it. On the one hand are your wallet and your time, both of which you are trying to protect – on the other, a team of very clever people, dedicated to separating you from both.

If you have a local butcher, fishmonger, baker, greengrocer – use them. In most instances they'll stock higher-quality products, and the shopping experience will be significantly more personal and less stressful. Ditto farmers' markets and specialist ethnic stores. Signing up for a regular vegetable/fruit box delivery can save you hassle while keeping you healthy – and expose you to foods you may not have tried before. Buying online and getting your groceries delivered will save you time, provided you don't linger on random products – and any extra fee (check out the annual passes that are sometimes available, since these often mean delivery is extremely cheap) is surely worth the chunk of afternoon you've saved.

Bargain supermarkets can save you money if you are prepared to shop creatively and can live with brands you've never heard of. Some may draw the line at ketchup, baked beans and teabags, where the staple brands set the bar high. Beware particularly the 'bargain' impulse buy here – if you set out to buy bread and cheese, but come home with a lawnmower and a bag of frozen kumquats, you have not saved money. For basic household items, toiletries etc, try super-cheap discount stores. Focus on what you came in for and do not be distracted by jumbo packs of sweets/candies.

If you do go to the supermarket in person, prepare yourself accordingly. Wising up to the incredible array of tricks employed to get you to spend more than you intended will mean you are able to resist them. Learn to read nutrition labels, write a shopping list, plan a route around the store. Do not shop hungry, or you will wind up with a trolley full of rubbish snack foods.

Planning

Start with a list, before you leave home, and aim to mostly stick to it. Give yourself a bit of freedom compiling it, but have a rough meal plan in mind – think about how many days you are buying for, ingredients for easy dishes, the nights you are likely to be out, when people are coming over. Keep a running list somewhere of basic items you are out of.

Supermarkets assault your senses with choice, including things you didn't know you needed, because you don't. Big brands pay extra for the right to be up in your face – for bargains look down, or up. Supermarkets deliberately don't put the stuff that everyone needs near the tills and exit, because they want you to linger. Stay focused. Write your list in the order you'll be walking around the store. Starting with fruit and veg is a good habit that encourages you to prioritise eating well. Look for produce that is in good shape, ripe or nearly ripe, with fragrance you can smell. Buying in season or local will help – if it's been shipped in from Peru, it is neither.

With supermarket offers, remember that it's only a bargain if it's something you are actually going to use. Watch for sell-by dates, especially on dairy/meat/fish. Usually the stuff with the longest shelf life will be at the

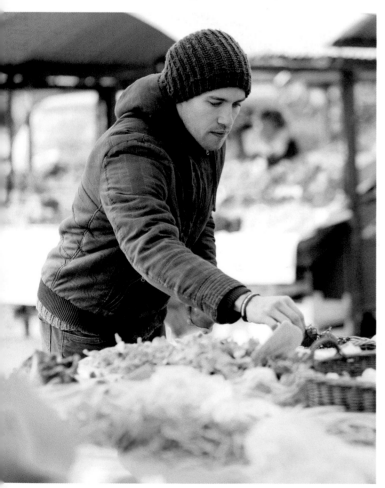

'A fruit is a vegetable with looks and money. Plus, if you let fruit rot, it turns into wine, something Brussels sprouts never do'
P. J. O'Rourke

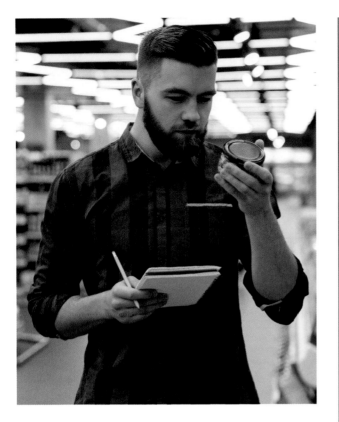

very back. As for seafood, if you live near the sea, find a local fishmonger and buy from them. Otherwise, frozen is fine – since much of the stuff on the fish counter will have been previously frozen and defrosted, there's little difference.

Reading nutrition labels

Beware foods that are marketed as healthy, but aren't. 'Fat-free' could apply to a bag of sugar, and a tub of lard can be labelled 'low-sugar'. Foods 'rich in Omega-3' may also be rich in salt and saturated fats. 'Organic' does not mean 'healthy'.

Pre-packaged foods come with nutrition labels – learn to read them and look out for the stuff that matters to your health. They will list information on how much energy is contained, in kilojoules (kj) or calories (kcal). Keep an eye on salt, fat, saturated fat, and sugars. These figures are usually expressed by serving and by a standard measure – eg 100g/4oz. Use this column to check between products, and find out if the 'healthy' granola is really just a big bowl of sugar that happens to be high in fibre.

Ingredients lists on the label give contents in order of their weight – so, if the first word is sugar, or salt, approach with care. Some products – depending on where you live – also have a label featuring colour-coded nutritional information, telling you if the food has high, medium or low amounts of fat, saturated fat, sugars and salt. Red = bad, green = good, yellow = in between.

Storing food

- ◆ Dry stuff – pasta etc – goes in the cupboard. Potatoes and some other veg – eg onions – live happily in a dark cupboard, but the fridge is also fine. Never ever store tomatoes in a fridge – it ruins the flavour. Ditto bananas.
- ◆ Meat, fish and dairy should be refrigerated, always. Butter left out is spreadable but will go rancid so it is best to slice off a small chunk to keep out and keep the rest of the packet wrapped in the fridge. Raw meat/poultry should always be kept separately, in clean sealed containers, on a separate shelf at the bottom of the fridge if possible.
- ◆ 'Use by' dates should be taken seriously, even if the food looks OK. Food poisoning is no fun. 'Best before' dates give a little more leeway.
- ◆ Many foods can be frozen. Cool it quickly, if just cooked, then wrap it in a sealed plastic bag or container so it doesn't dry out or absorb flavours from other foods. It won't last forever – if it looks grey/dry when thawed, don't eat it.
- ◆ Always defrost meat or fish properly before cooking/eating – best left overnight in the fridge.
- ◆ Don't put hot food in the fridge or freezer – it warms up everything else. Let a dish made for storage cool before chilling. The food, not you.
- ◆ Buy a load of freezer-proof plastic containers (or wash and keep the tub when you've scoffed all the ice cream or takeaway curry) and resealable freezer bags – batch cooking and freezing is the best habit to form.
- ◆ For covering leftovers in the fridge and when reheating foods, invest in some soft silicone food covers and suction lids that can go in the microwave and the oven. These mean you don't have to keep using cling film and foil, both of which are not great for the environment.

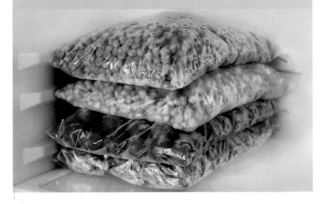

KITCHEN SKILLS

If you are starting from scratch, the best way to build confidence in the kitchen is by focusing on acquiring a few key skills. The man who can cook perfect rice, chop an onion and use a knife is well equipped for any culinary challenge – because the techniques you pick up in mastering these basics can be applied to almost any meal.

Read the recipe

This may seem bleedingly obvious, but nevertheless: before cooking from a recipe, read the whole thing through, carefully. Check you have the right amounts of all the ingredients (or acceptable substitutes), that you understand instructions/measurements/techniques, and don't start making something that needs a food processor if you don't own a food processor. Follow the recipe as closely as you can the first time, after which you can start to freestyle.

Knife skills

If you spend money and time on one kitchen item (other than a good pan) make it the knife. Learning different techniques can help you save time, and gives off a confident, cheffy vibe that's bound to impress.

Grip

Grasp the handle of the knife in a way that feels natural and keeps stray fingers out of the line of fire. Many beginner cooks are more comfortable wrapping the whole of the hand around the handle, behind the bolster (the bit that separates the blade and handle) but you will get more control with a blade grip – whereby the forefinger and thumb pinch either side of the blade.

Chop

Cut the foodstuff to make one side flat, so it rests securely on the chopping board. Use your non-knife hand to hold the food steady, knuckles curled under to keep your fingers out of the way. Position the knife on the food, resting the flat of the blade against your hand. Press down, smoothly and firmly, letting the sharpness of the blade do the work, pushing slightly forwards for momentum and to ready you to repeat the stroke.

Slice

Ready food and knife as above. Place the tip of the knife on the board and draw it towards you through the food. As it enters and slices, push down on the handle and slightly forwards to finish the slice. The knife stays in contact with the board throughout.

Mince

For herbs, garlic and other ingredients you want to mince finely, use a curved blade and a flat surface. Place the knife on the ingredients and grip the knife as above. Place your other hand on the top of the tip of the knife and rock the blade like a see-saw, making sure it always stays in contact with the chopping board.

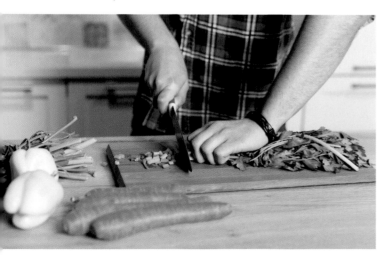

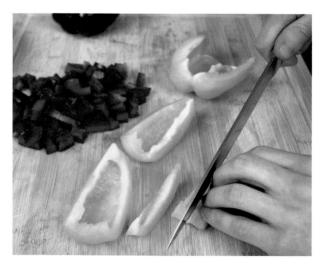

HOW TO
FINELY CHOP AN ONION

Many of the world's best dishes start with an onion – becoming efficient with your chopping technique will save you time and effort.

Equipment
Knife, chopping board.

1 Peel the onion, cutting off the top. Cut in half vertically. Place one half flat side down on the board and hold each side with your thumb and fingers make a bridge.

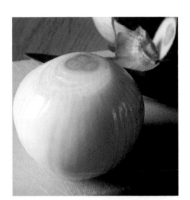

2 Chopping under the bridge of your fingers, use the knife to make cuts the length of the onion, from just before the root to the tip.

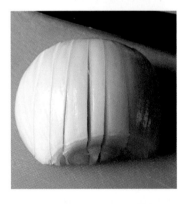

3 Then turn the onion round a quarter turn and still holding each side slice at right angles to the first cuts until just before the root end. Discard the root end.

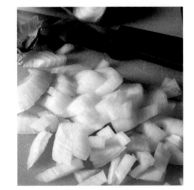

Tip
To 'roughly' chop just follow steps 1 and 2 but cut thicker slices, and don't follow up with the second stage of cutting. Onions take time to cook properly – if the recipe says 'cook until soft', it will take about 15 minutes. If you need to also soften garlic, give the onion a good head start before adding the garlic, otherwise it will burn before the onion softens.

Cooking terms

Relatively easy recipes can seem more daunting when they throw in terms that assume you already know the difference between a béchamel and bread sauce.

Baste:	Spoon liquid over the outside of a food that is being roasted.
Beat:	Stir ingredients vigorously until smooth.
Whisk:	Beat ingredients with a whisk or fork, introducing air, to make them fluffy.
Boil:	Cook in water that is 100°C/212°F – ie that is bubbling vigorously.
Simmer:	Cook gently on a low heat, so that it bubbles lightly.
Al dente:	'To the tooth' – pasta that is slightly undercooked, to give it bite.
Blanch:	Immerse briefly in boiling water.
Blend:	Mix together two ingredients.
Braise:	Cook by sautéing in fat then simmering slowly in a little liquid.
Cream:	Beat together sugar and butter until soft and creamy.
Drizzle:	Lightly trickle liquid or sauce over a dish.
Fillet:	A boneless cut (fish or meat).
Fold:	Use a rubber spatula or wire whisk to gently combine light ingredients with a heavier mixture by lifting and stirring.
Grease:	Lubricate the inside of a pan with an oil or fat to stop food from sticking.
Marinate:	Leave meat or fish to soak in a sauce (marinade) before cooking.
Sauté:	Cook in a pan with a little oil or fat over a low heat.
Poach:	Cook gently in a liquid that is simmering.
Reduce:	'Cook down' a sauce by cooking over a fairly high heat and stirring until it thickens.
Simmer:	Cook at a temperature lower than boiling – typically, the sauce or liquid will bubble gently, but the bubbles will not pop.
Steam:	Cook using ingredients in a steamer or basket above boiling water in a lidded pan.
Whisk:	Beat food with a whisk to aerate.

HOW TO
COOK PASTA

Soggy pasta is the hallmark of the poor cook. Aim for al dente (with bite) by cooking for the very minimum time indicated on the packet (if it says 10 minutes, try 9). Test by scooping out a piece, letting it cool slightly, then biting it. A visible white core means it is underdone and needs a minute more before you test it again. Once it is ready, drain it immediately, reserving a spoonful or two of the pasta water, which can then be added to the sauce to help keep it loose.

Kitchen tips and fixes

- ◆ Out-of-date salad can be cooked (so long as it hasn't gone slimy). Fry it with oil and add it to pasta.
- ◆ Many herbs can be frozen fresh. Simply remove the leaves from the stalks, if applicable, put them in a freezer-proof bag and use as required.
- ◆ Parmesan rind can be chucked whole into a soup or risotto for added flavour (remove it before serving).
- ◆ A squeeze of lemon juice just before serving adds zing to almost any meal.
- ◆ It is best to use unsalted butter for cooking, especially baking, since it gives you control over the amount of salt in the finished dish. Some people prefer salted butter for putting on things, such as toast or baked potatoes.
- ◆ Too salty? Cancel it out by bulking it up (eg adding pasta to a soup) or by adding fats (butter, oil) or sharp flavours (lemon, vinegar). In extreme situations, drain and chuck some of the liquid and replace with something less salty…
- ◆ Too spicy? Add dairy – yogurt, cream, etc. Sweetness also works – try adding mango chutney to a curry to mellow it.
- ◆ Too greasy? Chuck in some ice cubes, leave them for about 30 seconds, then fish them out – the ice sticks to the fat. This is also a great way to remove the fat from the juices when roasting meat, before you turn it into gravy.
- ◆ Overcooked veg? Blend for a stylish purée – pretend it's what you meant to do. You could add a splash of cream or stir through some crème fraîche for a super-impressive side.
- ◆ Lumpy gravy? Pass it through a sieve, or whizz it with a stick blender.

HOW TO
COOK RICE

Rice is as easy to get wrong but the basic principles are the same: one standard mug full of uncooked rice will feed three to four people. Use twice the amount of water to rice.

Equipment
Mug, sieve, heavy pan with a lid, fork, clean tea towel.

1 Rinse one mug of rice in a sieve under running water – some rice also benefits from a soak.

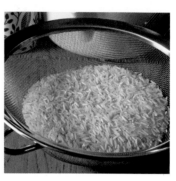

2 Melt a small knob of butter in a heavy pan with a lid, add the rice and stir to coat. Add two mugs of water and a pinch of salt.

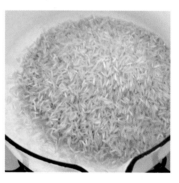

3 When the water bubbles stir once, turn the heat way down and stick on a well-fitting pan lid. After 10 minutes, check that the water has been absorbed and the grains are sticking up. The rice is now cooked.

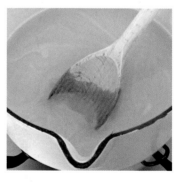

4 Fluff the rice up with a fork then drape a (clean) tea towel over it. Serve straight from the pan or transfer to a warm bowl for extra fluff.

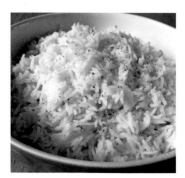

HOW TO
ROAST VEGETABLES

This is a quick and easy base for many main courses, soups, sauces and sides. Wash and chop a load of veg, stick them in a roasting tray, drizzle generously with olive oil, throw in garlic cloves, roast in the oven.

Serves 2

Ingredients
- 4 red, yellow or orange bell peppers, seeded and cut in to large chunks
- 2 medium sweet potatoes, peeled and diced
- 2 red onions, peeled and thickly sliced
- 1 fennel bulb
- olive oil
- 1 sprig fresh sage
- 3–4 sprigs fresh thyme or rosemary
- balsamic vinegar (optional)
- salt and ground black pepper

Method

1 Preheat the oven to 200°C/400°F/Gas 6. Cut the fronds, base and stalks from the bulb of fennel. Cut in half and slice thickly.

2 Tip all the vegetables into a roasting pan large enough for everything to be in a single layer. Pour in a good amount of olive oil, add plenty of salt and pepper and toss. Place the herbs on top. Roast for 20–30 minutes. Toss and turn halfway through the cooking time.

3 When the vegetables are tender and slightly charred in places, remove from the oven and add a drizzle of balsamic vinegar.

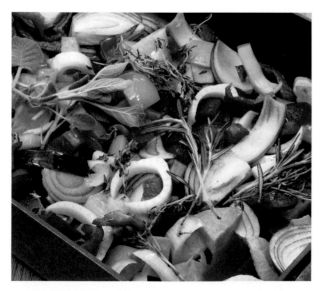

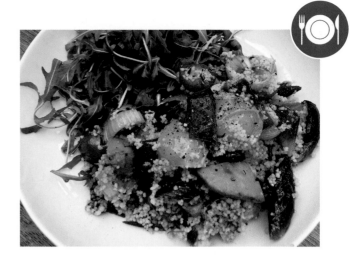

Serving suggestions
- Transfer to a pan, add chopped fresh tomatoes and 1 litre/1¾ pints/2 cups vegetable stock. Simmer for 20 minutes, then blend for a delicious soup.
- Mix with couscous and cubes of feta, sprinkle with toasted pine nuts and serve with rocket/arugula salad.
- Add a portion of ultimate tomato sauce (see recipe on p40) and serve with pasta, topped with grated Parmesan cheese.

HOW TO
MAKE A SALAD DRESSING

A well-dressed salad adds a professional and healthy touch to home-cooked meals. A dressing can be as simple as just oil and vinegar (add three parts of the former to one of the latter for a classic vinaigrette) but there is plenty of room for riffing with other ingredients, once you've got the basic recipe down. Here's mine:

Ingredients
- 30ml/2 tbsp red wine vinegar or balsamic vinegar
- 30ml/2 tbsp white wine vinegar
- 100ml/6 tbsp olive oil
- 10ml/2 tsp Dijon mustard
- 5ml/1 tsp clear honey or caster sugar
- generous pinch of sea salt and ground black pepper

Method

Combine all of the ingredients in a bowl and stir vigorously to blend, or place them in a screw-top jar and shake well. This keeps in the fridge for days so it's a good idea to make double the quantity.

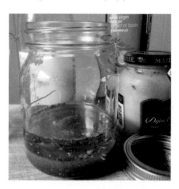

EVERYDAY EATING

What a man eats when he is alone is up to him – which is both liberating and terrifying. There may be a part of you rejoicing at this freedom and planning a lifetime of ketchup sandwiches. This is your inner child, and you can keep him happy with a diet of cookies and fries, if you choose (good luck with the diabetes). Or you can man up. Accepting full responsibility for your diet is a very good first step towards being grown up.

Getting started

It helps to be realistic. Know your culinary abilities, how much time and money you have, the extent to which you can be bothered, and start with meals that fit around those plans. If you are just learning to cook, begin with the basics and build from there. Once you can make a risotto, a pasta sauce, a curry and a soup you are well on the road to self-sufficiency – and ahead of many men.

There are a couple of essential recipes here to get you going, but you can't beat a good cookbook, magazine, blog

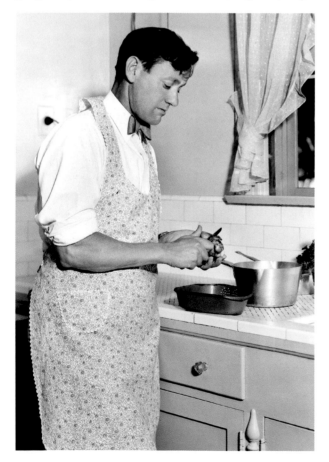

or cooking website for inspiration and advice, and of course you can always ask friends and family for their recipes if you've enjoyed eating something – they'll be flattered.

There are millions of recipes out there, suitable for different diets, budgets and abilities, as well as tastes. The sheer range of choice may make finding recipes seem a bit daunting, but really all you need to do is write down a list of the dishes you enjoy eating and want to make and then search online. Another approach is to search by entering in a few ingredients – ones that you really want to try out, or even just need to use before they go off – and see what comes up and floats your boat.

Checking out blogs and social media is a great way to follow cooks you like – who may not have written cookbooks – and get updated on a regular basis. You should, however, be aware that the recipes may not have been as rigorously tested before they are published as ones that appear in cookbooks and on more regulated websites, so it's often worth reading some of the comments to see what feedback is being given by people who've tried out the dishes – and what tweaks may work.

Collate recipes that you like the look of, wherever you find them, in an app such as Pocket, Pinterest or similar (or just bookmark them) and you'll soon find that you've created a personalised bank of reliable dishes that you can edit and add to at whim.

Whichever route you go for, be sure to check what measurements are used, since these differ from country to country: Australian cup measures are not the same as US ones, for instance. Whatever system you choose – metric, Imperial or cups – stick to that format for the whole recipe; don't suddenly switch halfway through.

When you are cooking for one you may not want to take hours over it, since the only person you are trying to impress is you. The aim is to create straightforward, delicious and nutritious meals, comprising a good mix of carbs, protein and vegetables. You may also be looking for economy, depending on your budget, and ideally a meal that can be eaten as leftovers tomorrow, or frozen for later. Conversely, recipes can be scaled down for one – use an online tool for adjusting measurements. It isn't necessary to buy in bulk – supermarket fish/meat counters will sell single portions if you don't have much freezer space.

Batch cooking

Many recipes can be scaled up and the leftovers saved for another day, making your life easier for very little extra effort. If you've got the time/inclination, you can devote an afternoon to doing a whole load of different recipes for the freezer. It takes a little organisation, but at some point in the future you will thank yourself. Top tips:

◆ Make sure you have enough containers, of the right size and shape – resealable freezer bags will do the job, or wash and reuse ice-cream containers and the like.
◆ Don't feel you have to slavishly double everything in the recipe – use your best judgement about spices and seasoning.
◆ Pretty much anything that cooks in a saucepan – a soup, stew, casserole – will freeze well.
◆ Don't overcook the food. You'll be giving it another blast of heat, and you don't want it turning to mush.
◆ Let the dish cool before freezing and make sure you write on the bag what it is, and when you made it – otherwise you will be staring at it in two months and wondering whether it is chilli or soup.

Seasoning

Added seasoning makes or breaks a dish – too little and it may be bland, too much, inedible. Generally, fresh herbs are best added at the end of the cooking process. For curries and other spice-based dishes, it is more usual to start by dry-frying them in a pan with no oil, to release the flavours. NB salt is not good for you, but it's why restaurant food tastes so good, so it's worth using just a little.

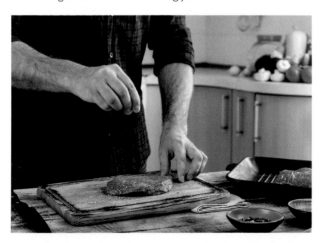

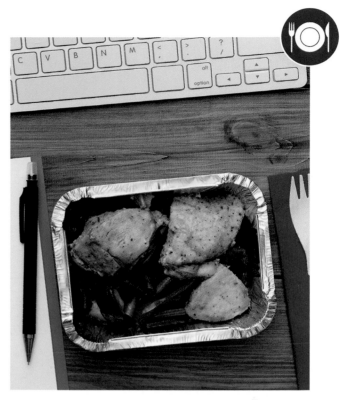

⋀ When you're planning an evening meal cook double quantities and save half for lunch the next day or freeze it for another evening when you're home late or the fridge is bare.

Love your leftovers

Don't throw away chicken bones. Pile them in a large pan, add an onion, a stick of celery, some chopped carrots and a sprig of fresh herbs and cover with water. Cover and bring to the boil, then turn down the heat and simmer for an hour or two. Drain the stock into a bowl and allow it to cool, then refrigerate if you have a plan for it, freeze if you don't. Some rainy day you'll cook some pasta in this and make chicken noodle soup.

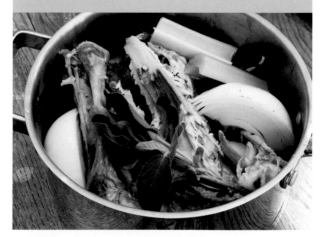

QUICK BREAKFASTS

Thinking about breakfast the night before will save you from running out of the house empty-bellied, and resorting to grabbing something unhealthy/expensive from a coffee shop or takeaway stall. You are aiming for slow-release energy that will keep you going through until lunch, which is why oats are your best friend. Cheap and nutritious, they can be endlessly customised.

Bircher muesli

Soaking the oats overnight breaks them down and means they become creamy without having to be cooked. Make it in a sealable plastic container to eat on the move.

Ingredients
- 50g/2oz/½ cup rolled oats
- 1 small apple, grated
- 50ml/2fl oz/¼ cup milk of your choice
- 15ml/1 tbsp natural/plain yogurt
- 15ml/1 tbsp sunflower seeds (optional)
- sliced banana, toasted nuts and seeds, dried fruit, fresh berries, extra yogurt or clear honey, to serve

Method
Place the oats in a small bowl, add the grated apple, milk and yogurt and mix well. Cover, or transfer to a clip-seal jar, and refrigerate overnight. Serve the soft oats with a topping of your choice.

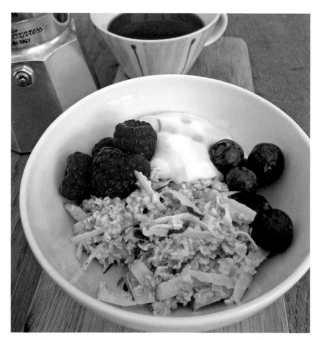

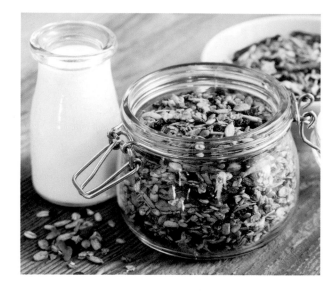

Home-made granola

This can be tweaked and improvised to suit what you like and what's in the cupboard. Seeds (and some nuts) are cheap, and deliver a huge nutrition boost.

Ingredients
- 300g/11oz/3 cups rolled oats
- 60ml/4 tbsp clear honey
- 1.25ml/¼ tsp each ground cinnamon and nutmeg
- 115g/4oz mixed chopped nuts and flaked almonds
- 50g/2oz/⅓ cup seeds – sunflower, sesame, whatever
- 60ml/4 tbsp rapeseed or other mild vegetable oil
- pinch of salt
- 115g/4oz/scant 1 cup raisins or dried cranberries
- milk or yogurt and fresh fruit, to serve

Method
1 Preheat the oven to 160°C/325°F/Gas 3. Mix together all the ingredients except the raisins in a large bowl. Scatter on to a baking tray (it needs to have sides) and cook for 30–40 minutes, stirring every 10 minutes.

2 Halfway through, add the raisins and give everything a good stir – the oats at the edges cook faster, so redistribute them around the pan. When crisp and golden remove from the oven and cool completely.

3 Transfer the granola to a sealed plastic container/glass jar and it'll keep for 2–3 weeks. Serve with milk or yogurt and fresh fruit.

HOW TO BE
YOUR OWN BARISTA

Happily for those who like to savour coffee there is an increasing market for carefully sourced and created brews – and many people spend hundreds on takeaway coffee every year. It's true that a great coffee shop will have a very good, very expensive espresso machine – and it is impossible to precisely replicate the pressure these generate – so specialist coffee shops definitely have their place. (NB always take your own reusable cup if you know you'll want a takeaway coffee – like not taking bags to the supermarket, it is totally irresponsible and no longer acceptable to constantly require disposable single-use cups that account for millions of tons of waste every year.) The art of making coffee is, however, relatively simple – it's all about extracting the flavour from the beans in a form that suits your tastes – and you can do that very well at home.

Start with good beans (buying single estate ones will enable you to more accurately control the end result, and will also educate your palate) and a grinder. Coffee begins to lose its flavour soon after it is ground and pulverising your beans as and when you want them not only produces the best results but is also satisfying and releases an intoxicating smell. Don't be tempted to misuse a blender you've previously used for something else – you want to taste only the coffee, not garlic.

There are an enormous number of coffee-making systems out there, but it isn't necessary to spend a fortune. Simple pour-over filter systems (the best are Japanese) offer an excellent cup at a low cost. More fiddly but equally effective are modern coffee presses, which use pressure, a rubber seal and elbow grease, and the classic stovetop espresso.

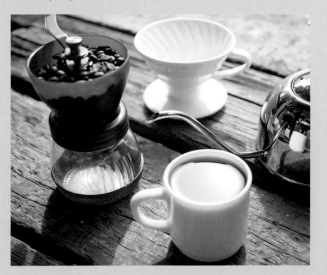

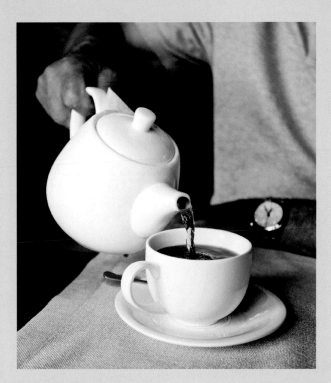

Don't forget tea

Chucking a teabag in a mug and sloshing over some boiling water is the most common, and convenient, method for making tea, but sometimes it's worth taking a little more care to elevate the everyday to the extraordinary.

1 Fill the kettle with fresh water; reboiling it produces a duller flavour.

2 Just before the kettle boils, pour a small amount of the water into the teapot and swill it around (carefully) for about 30 seconds to warm it. Tip away the water.

3 Put your tea of choice into the pot – the rule of thumb is about 5ml/1 tsp loose-leaf tea per person plus one for the pot, or two teabags for a standard-size teapot, depending on how strong you like it.

4 At exactly the moment the kettle boils, pour water into the pot and leave to brew for up to 7 minutes for loose-leaf tea, and about 3½ minutes for teabags.

5 Pour the tea into a fine teacup if possible (or a clean mug, if not). Pour through a strainer if using loose-leaf. Add milk and sugar as liked, put your feet up and savour.

WEEKEND BREAKFASTS

Brunch

If you work Monday to Friday, your weekday breakfast may be a rushed affair. Which is why one of the great pleasures of the weekend is a leisurely late breakfast on your own, or brunch with friends. True, this can be particularly enjoyable when someone else is doing the cooking, but if you learn to recreate the expensive options available in hipster joints you will thank yourself – not only for the enormous amount of money you save, but for the lack of time queuing and the guarantee that everything will be cooked exactly as you like it. And the joy of eating in your pjs.

To knock your socks off, a brunch has to comprise the very best ingredients – fresh coffee or top-quality tea, free-range eggs, tomatoes that taste of something, fresh bread. If you are going for an old-school fry-up then there's a lot of guilty pleasure to be gained from a supermarket sausage – but if you've got a good butcher, you'll taste the difference and its likely to contain slightly less junk, too.

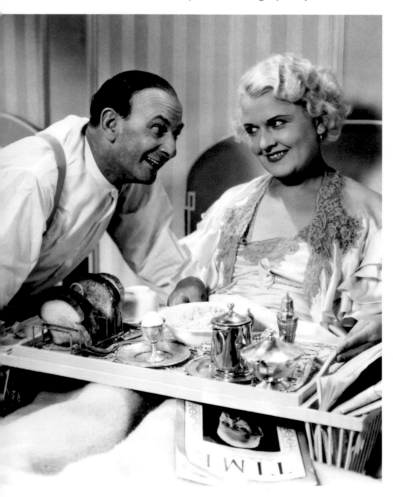

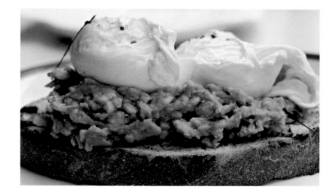

Avocado toast

This nutritious treat is incredibly easy to rustle up – the only tricky part is finding avocados that are suitably ripe.

Serves 2

Ingredients

- 1 ripe avocado
- 5ml/1 tsp lemon juice
- 2 pieces hot sourdough toast
- finely sliced seeded red chilli (optional)
- salt and ground black pepper
- 2 poached or soft boiled eggs, to serve

Method

Halve the avocado, remove the pit and scoop out the flesh. Mash in a bowl with lemon juice and seasoning. Spread the avocado mixture on the hot toast and sprinkle over the chilli. Top with a poached egg.

Variation

Spread cream cheese on the toast, lay slices of avocado on top, then sprinkle over salt, smoked paprika or cayenne pepper, and a squeeze of lemon juice.

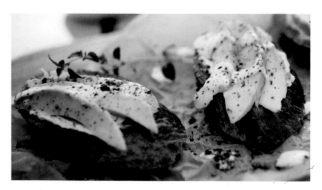

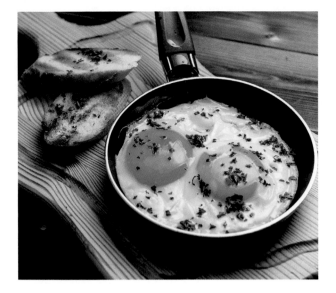

Fried eggs on toast

It can seem a fair amount of hassle when you're bleary eyed, but an egg provides a great protein hit at the start of the day, and is packed with vitamins and minerals. There are lots of way to cook them – poached, scrambled, boiled – but fried eggs are possibly the easiest and quickest. There are various methods out there: this is mine.

Serves 1

Ingredients
◆ 2.5ml/½ tsp oil – light olive oil is good
◆ 2 eggs
◆ buttered toast and condiments, to serve

Method

1 Place a non-stick pan over a medium-high heat and, when hot, add the oil. Once the oil is hot, crack in the eggs, taking care not to break the yolks.

2 Cook the eggs for about 4 minutes, or until the whites are just opaque all the way through. Flip the egg briefly if prefer the yolk to be more cooked, or serve sunny side up.

3 Serve with buttered toast and the condiment of your choice – sriracha gives a good spicy kick.

Stuffed French toast

A cooked breakfast is the best way to start the weekend, if someone else is doing the clearing up, but it does involve fine timing and a lot of multi-tasking. For a more relaxed brunch, try French toast. Served with maple syrup and bacon it makes a great substitute for pancakes, or you can sandwich it together with cream cheese and fruit, as here.

Ingredients
◆ handful of blueberries, washed and dried
◆ 15ml/1 tbsp roasted chopped hazelnuts
◆ drizzle of maple syrup or clear honey
◆ 4 thick slices of brioche or white bread
◆ cream cheese
◆ 1 egg
◆ splash of milk
◆ light vegetable oil, for frying
◆ pat of butter
◆ caster/superfine sugar, for sprinkling

Method

1 Mix together the blueberries with the hazelnuts and maple syrup or honey.

2 Lay the slices of brioche or bread on a board and spread two of them thickly with cream cheese. Add the blueberries and hazelnuts in a single layer on top.

3 Spread the other slices of brioche less thickly with cream cheese and then use to top the slices covered with the berry mixture, pressing down to seal. You should now have two sandwiches.

4 Mix together the egg and milk in a wide, shallow dish. Heat the oil in a frying pan on a medium heat – it needs to be hot before anything goes in.

5 Dip both sides of the sandwiches in the beaten egg and transfer to the hot pan. Cook both sides for 3–4 minutes or until golden brown. When the second sides are almost done, add a pat of butter to the pan for a luxurious finish, turning the sandwiches over to coat both sides. Remove from the pan and sprinkle the tops generously with sugar. Serve immediately, while hot and crispy.

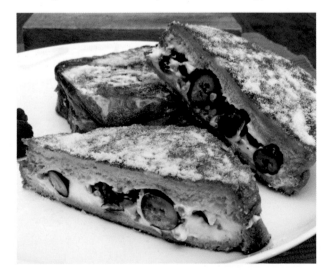

EASY LUNCHES

After breakfast, lunch is the second-greatest nutritional black hole in a man's life. Too many guys rely on supermarket sandwiches, which seem harmless until you read the nutrition label – even upmarket butties can contain shocking amounts of salt and fat.

By far the easiest lunch is leftover dinner from the night before. Many foods become even more delicious for having been left to their own devices for a while – curry, chilli, soup can mellow and release subtle flavours the next day. Make it a habit to double the ingredients when cooking dinner and put the spare portion on a plate or in a suitable container, ready for reheating or transporting.

The art of the sandwich

We don't have to tell you how to make a sandwich – the skill here lies in the creative choice of filling and condiments. Use the best bread you can, on nutritional and taste grounds – crusty rolls or a French stick will be less prone to sogginess. Toasting the bread/buttering it before filling it also works. Stock your fridge with interesting sauces, pickles, chutneys, etc to bring interest to a cheese roll. Put sandwiches in a plastic container of a suitable size if possible, or use a plastic sandwich bag or wrap it tightly in foil.

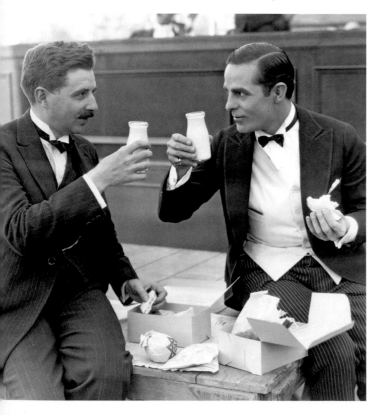

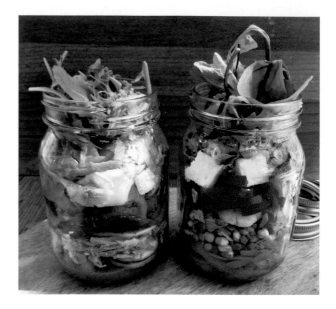

Mason jar salad

Jar salads are a great invention – because the dressing stays at the bottom, none of the salad spoils, meaning you can prepare it the evening before. If you have a punishing commute, swap the heavy glass for a lighter sealable plastic container instead. Mix and match with whatever you have in the fridge/cupboard, following the principles below.

1 Start with a good portion of salad dressing at the bottom of the jar, making sure there is enough to dress the whole jarful and it is well seasoned with salt and pepper.

2 Next, add a layer of robust vegetables that will benefit from marinating in the dressing: roasted root vegetables, sliced fennel or courgette/zucchini, shredded cabbage.

3 The next layers should be tender vegetables such as sprouting seeds, peas, corn, sliced red bell peppers, followed by protein – chicken, ham or tuna, prawns/shrimp or smoked salmon, sliced hard-boiled egg, cubes of tofu – then (cooked) carbs, such as noodles, pasta or rice.

4 Add some cheese and more fragile vegetables such as tomato, cucumber, spinach and salad leaves. Pack it down before adding leaves so you can fit lots in.

5 Screw or clip on the lid and refrigerate. To serve, tip into a bowl or plate. If eating straight from the jar, give it a good shake first to disperse the dressing.

HOW TO
MAKE AN OMELETTE

A man who can make an omelette can cook himself a meal, from common kitchen ingredients, that works at any time of the day. It is also ready in less than 10 minutes. Fillings are up to you; sautéed mushrooms, pulled ham, roasted tomatoes, cold chicken, goat's cheese and herbs…

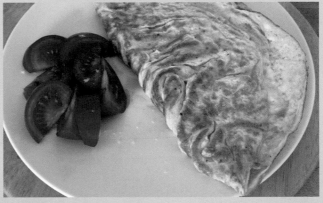

Ingredients
- ◆ 2–3 large (US extra large) eggs
- ◆ 15ml/1 tbsp milk
- ◆ 10ml/2 tsp butter or olive oil
- ◆ handful of grated cheese
- ◆ salt and ground black pepper

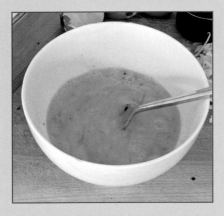

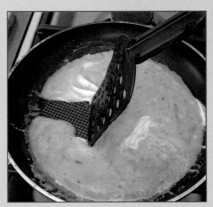

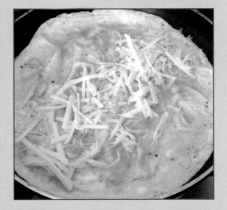

1 Crack the eggs into a small bowl, add a splash of milk, salt and some ground black pepper. Beat with a fork until mixed. Grate the cheese and set aside. Place a small non-stick frying pan over a medium heat and add the butter or oil.

2 When the butter is foaming or bubbling, pour in the beaten egg. As it begins to set, use a spatula to pull in the sides of the omelette and tilt the pan so that you get soft folds in the egg.

3 When the omelette is starting to firm up, sprinkle over the cheese. Then, when golden underneath and the egg on top is just cooked, use the spatula to fold it in half, and slide it on to a plate. Serve immediately.

Variations

Omelettes are easily adapted. Try adding some baby spinach leaves on top of the cheese, they will wilt when you fold it over. Shredded ham or salami with cubes of feta cheese and fresh tomato turns a breakfast dish into a quick supper, while sautéed mushrooms and a dash of cream makes a more substantial meal for any time of the day served with bread and salad.

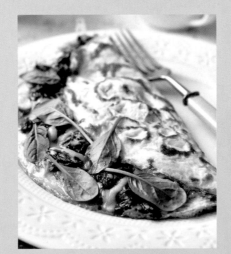

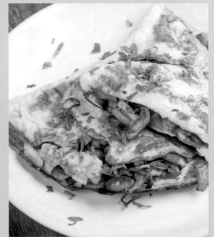

DINNER FOR ONE

Dining alone need not feel tragic. The focus is on pleasing yourself, whether this means economy, speed, or enjoying a potter around the kitchen cooking for pleasure.

Ultimate tomato sauce

This tomato sauce is the single man's saviour, perfect for portioning up and freezing for later use. It is delicious with pasta, couscous, polenta or rice, can be turned into soup, used for a pizza topping, or added to roasted veg.

Makes 4 portions

Ingredients
- 3 onions, peeled and finely chopped
- 3 garlic cloves, peeled and minced
- 15ml/1 tbsp sugar
- about 300ml/½ pint/1¼ cups vegetable stock
- 4 x 400g/14oz cans tomatoes
- 120ml/4 tbsp tomato paste
- glug of olive oil
- generous splash of balsamic vinegar
- Seasonings to taste: salt, herbs (dried oregano or fresh basil), chilli flakes

Method

1 Heat the oil in a very large pan over a medium heat, then add the onions, reduce the heat and sweat down, stirring occasionally, for about 10 minutes. Add the garlic and continue to sweat for a further 5 minutes.

2 Stir in the sugar, tomatoes and tomato paste and simmer for about 30–45 minutes, until reduced. Season to taste and add a splash of balsamic vinegar.

3 Leave to cool, then divide into four equal portions and transfer to freezer bags for defrosting as needed.

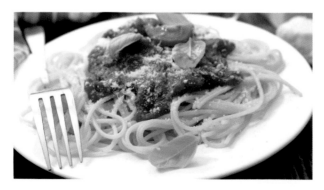

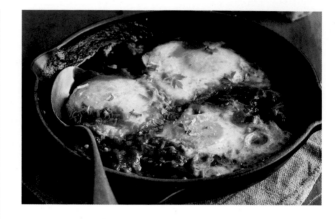

Shakshuka

Use a portion of ultimate tomato sauce to create shakshuka, a North African dish that makes a great weekend breakfast or a quick and easy supper for one.

Serves 1

Ingredients
- 1 red bell pepper, seeded and sliced
- 1 onion, peeled and finely sliced
- 15ml/1 tbsp olive oil
- 2.5ml/½ tsp smoked paprika
- pinch each of cayenne pepper and ground cumin
- 1 portion of ultimate tomato sauce
- 2 or 3 eggs (4 if you're feeding two)
- handful of fresh coriander/cilantro
- salt and ground black pepper

Method

1 Heat the olive oil in a frying pan over a medium heat, then add the pepper and onion and cook gently for about 15 minutes, until soft. Stir in the spices. Add the tomato sauce and simmer for 5–10 minutes, until reduced and thick. If you don't have any sauce made up, use a 400g/14oz can of tomatoes and simmer for 20 minutes.

2 When the sauce is thickened, taste and season with salt and pepper if necessary. Make little dents, crack an egg into each and turn the heat to low. Cover with a lid and cook for 5–10 minutes until the eggs are just set.

3 Sprinkle over some chopped coriander and carefully transfer the mixture to a bowl, without breaking the eggs, or eat it from the pan with crusty bread.

HOW TO
COOK THE PERFECT STEAK

The principles of cooking any cut of steak are basically the same. Start by pan-frying thick fillet steak/beef tenderloin, which is probably the most forgiving cut and the easiest to get right. Get the butcher to cut 4cm/1½ inch-thick steaks for the following instructions.

Equipment
Cast-iron frying pan or griddle, tongs.

Cooking times

For blue (very rare) steak, cook it for 1½ minutes on each side. For rare, 2½ minutes each side; for medium, 4 minutes each side; and for a well-done steak cook for 5 minutes each side. Use a stopwatch or kitchen timer for exact cooking times.

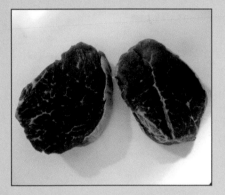

1 Store the steaks in the fridge, but remove and bring to room temperature before cooking. This helps to tenderise the meat. Heat a cast-iron frying pan, griddle or the best frying pan you own on a high heat.

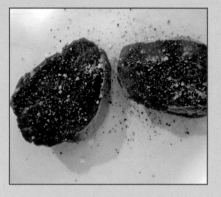

2 Just before you cook the steak, sprinkle one side with salt and ground black pepper (don't do this until just before you cook, or the salt will start to draw out moisture).

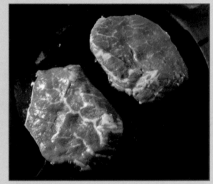

3 Add a little oil to the hot pan and when it's smoking, place the steaks, seasoned side down, into the pan – they should start to sizzle instantly.

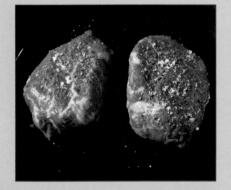

4 Set a timer for 2½ minutes. Just before the time is up, season the top of the steaks with pepper and salt, then turn them over using tongs.

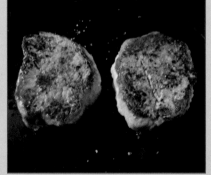

5 Cook the second side of the steak for another 2½ minutes. This timing will give you a medium-rare steak.

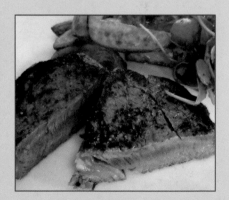

6 Remove the steaks from the pan and leave to rest for at least 5 minutes before serving with accompaniments and condiments of your choice. A simple green salad and some oven-roasted potatoes or crisp French fries are ideal.

SUCCESSFUL ENTERTAINING

Sooner or later you are going to have to have people round, otherwise you'll never be invited back and will live a lonely life. Begin with a simple drinks party with easy nibbles and bought in finger food, work up to cooking for someone other than yourself. If this is a new or daunting experience, fear not – the truth is, you can bluff your way to making others believe you are a great cook with relatively little effort. Focus on creating the right atmosphere and providing two or three well-chosen dishes, add in some creative presentation and a generous pouring hand and the job is done. A big part of the success of any evening at home is the attitude of the host. Be genial, be laid-back, pretend you care less than you do, and don't let a burned steak stress you out.

Have a plan

Plan ahead. Know what you are going to cook, and practise it on yourself. Keep it simple, doable, but with a little flourish – and with as much of the hard work as possible done in advance. There are some dishes that impress on a plate but can actually take little effort to cook – fish, for instance. Preparing an appetiser in addition to the main and dessert elevates home cooking instantly, as does serving a creative side or salad. If three courses feels overwhelming, there is no shame at all in cheating – no one will complain if you serve a bought-in dessert.

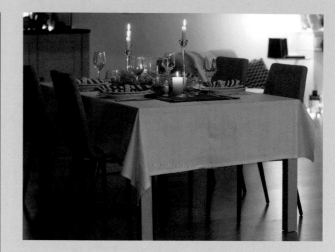

▲ Getting the ambience right is at least as important as the food.

Atmosphere

Job number one: get the vibe right. For dude night, this might mean not much more than putting the TV on and making sure there is sufficient beer. For a date, it will involve setting the table properly and considering music and lighting choices. Candles are an instant win (be sure not to burn the house down) and lamps will always be better than a bright overhead light. Prepare a playlist, either of digital music or by setting out in your mind what you want to play. Obviously make the place as tidy and clean as you can, including those areas you don't imagine a guest will see. While we are on presentation, don't neglect yourself – dress after any messy kitchen stuff has happened, but before the guests arrive. And wear an apron – it protects your clothes and says you know what you're doing, even if you don't.

Prep

Job number two: do as much prep work as you can before anyone arrives. You don't want to be spending the evening in the kitchen while a guest is left to their own devices in the other room. Above all, be ready to put a drink – alcoholic or soft – in the guest's hand when they walk through the door. A mixed cocktail (or mocktail) chilled, in a jug and ready to pour (prepare the glasses too – ideally the right ones for the drink) will get you off to a flying start, as will some chilled fizz.

Whatever your tipple, be sure it is an upgrade on the usual – a particularly good/unusual wine or decent craft beer makes for a talking point. Small bowls of nibbles take the pressure off the cook and give you an opportunity to hang with guests, being polite, before you disappear to do any last-minute kitchen stuff.

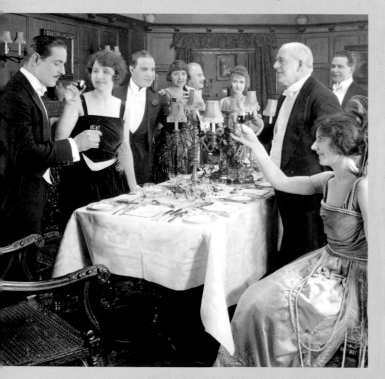

Setting a table

Half of the secret of entertaining is presentation. If you want to serve a truly classy dinner, you will need posh plates, posh cutlery and posh glassware – and an idea of where to put them. If you don't own these, then just using your usual stuff properly will make all the difference.

◆ Start by laying a tablecloth if you have one, with placemats on top for each setting.
◆ Lay out the plate for the main course. Put it in the centre of whatever placemat you are using.
◆ Cutlery goes in the order in which it will be used, from the outside in.

◆ Forks go to the left, knives and spoons to the right. Fork prongs face the ceiling, knife edges face the plate. Cutlery for desserts goes above the plate, with the spoon pointing left and the fork, if applicable, pointing right.
◆ Salad or appetizer plates, or soup bowls can be placed on top of the dinner plate, bread plates go top left of the setting.
◆ A folded or rolled napkin, if you have them, goes on the left hand side of the setting, you can also place it on the plate if you're short of space.
◆ Put a red wine glass and a white wine glass to the upper right of the plate, and add a tumbler for water.

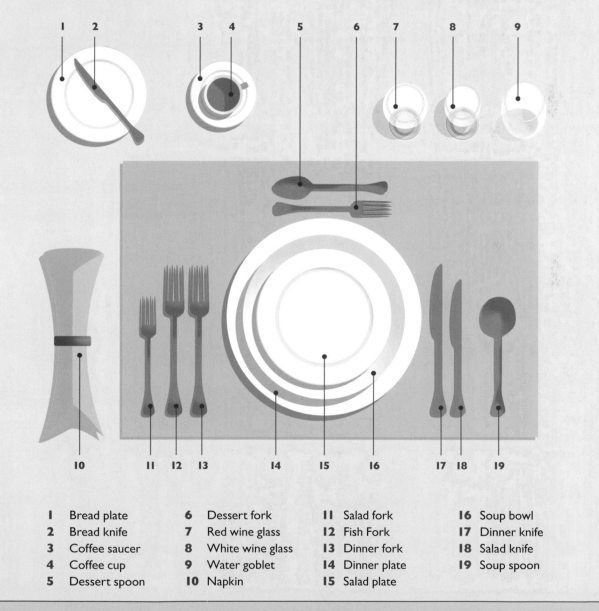

1 Bread plate	**6** Dessert fork	**11** Salad fork	**16** Soup bowl
2 Bread knife	**7** Red wine glass	**12** Fish Fork	**17** Dinner knife
3 Coffee saucer	**8** White wine glass	**13** Dinner fork	**18** Salad knife
4 Coffee cup	**9** Water goblet	**14** Dinner plate	**19** Soup spoon
5 Dessert spoon	**10** Napkin	**15** Salad plate	

IMPRESS A DATE

There comes a moment in every man's life when he meets someone he wishes to impress. You've demonstrated your mastery of manners in the restaurant, proved yourself worthy on the dance floor, rolled out the charm for their friends and family. But you haven't shown yourself at your fullest – a capable modern man – until they've seen what you can do in the kitchen.

What you are demonstrating here is the range of qualities that make you an ideal partner. You are showing you can provide, the cornerstone of man's appeal since your ancestors braved countless hazards to drag home woolly mammoth fillets for dinner. The fact you only went as far as the supermarket fish counter is neither here nor there – you are showing you have the means, the skills and the inclination to care for another person, and that's a biggie.

Stay cool. You are aiming to provide a great meal without letting the effort show – your reputation for competence will be severely dented if you freak out about a burned pine nut. Laugh at your mistakes, and be ready to serve a sandwich if it all goes wrong.

Start early, and leave time to get yourself and the whole place ready. Make sure the lighting, music and mood are set – and all your food prep is done. You want to look like a TV chef, with ready chopped ingredients to hand and all the difficult stuff done in advance. Prepare a welcome drink – if you know your date's favourite, serve that. If you don't, find

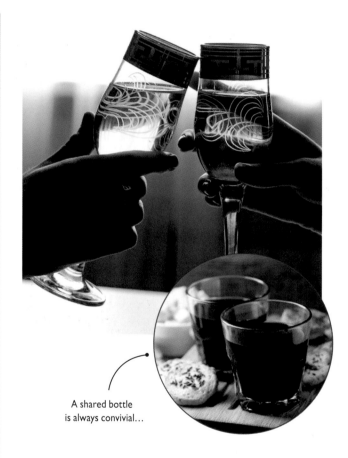

A shared bottle is always convivial…

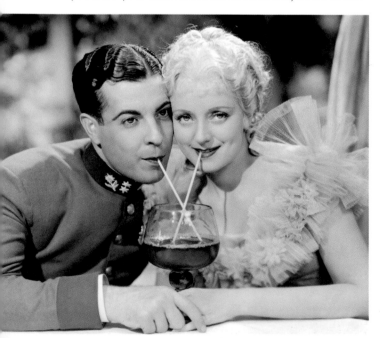

out, and if you can't, play it safe with fizz and have a soft drink to hand as a back-up. Champagne, prosecco or Cava are all fine – buy the best you can afford, and make sure it is as chilled as you are. TIP: Placing the bottle in a bucket of iced water will chill it quicker than ice alone.

Three courses will impress mightily, but two will certainly do the job. Avoid very rich or garlicky food (there may not be kissing later, but why jinx yourself?) Do what you can to learn about your guest's food preferences – you don't want to find out they are gluten-free as you serve the pizza, or veggie as you carve the roast. Above all, do not attempt something you've never cooked before. Road-test it on yourself, if necessary – preferably a few days before.

Appetiser

Go for an easy appetiser – something store-bought that takes only a little pimping on your part is ideal, or a dish that can be prepped way in advance, such as the pâté given here.

Smoked mackerel pâté

A variation on the Italian antipasti platter, this is a quick first course that impresses with little effort. Be inspired by what's available at the fishmonger/deli counter, and go for gravadlax, soused herring, potted shrimp or dressed crab. Whatever you buy in, make this home-made pâté your centrepiece – it is impressive and ridiculously easy.

Serves 4

Ingredients

◆ 2 smoked mackerel fillets
◆ 30ml/2 tbsp cream cheese
◆ 5–10ml/1–2 tsp creamed horseradish
◆ juice of 1 lemon
◆ black pepper
◆ cayenne pepper, to garnish

Method

1 Peel the skins from the mackerel fillets and discard, then flake the flesh into a mixing bowl, removing any bones as you do so. Add the cream cheese and horseradish, half the lemon juice and a good grinding of black pepper.

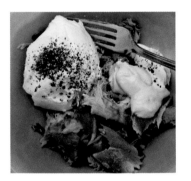

2 Using a fork, mash the fish into the cream cheese until well combined, and you have achieved the texture you prefer; keep going for a really smooth pâté. Taste, and add more lemon juice, pepper or horseradish if needed. Cover and refrigerate for 1–2 hours so the flavours can develop.

3 When ready to serve, scoop into one or two smaller bowls and dust with a little cayenne pepper, then arrange on a board with smoked salmon, prawns, lemon wedges and Scandinavian crispbreads.

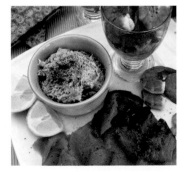

Easy antipasti

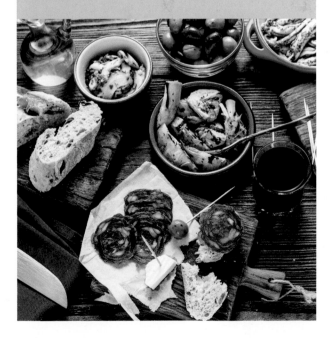

A large platter of antipasti is a great way to start any kind of supper or dinner party. It works well as an informal, help-yourself appetiser that can be expanded to serve large numbers, or as nibbles you and your guest can pick at while you cook the main course. Get it ready in advance, then cover with a clean cloth.

Take inspiration from the deli counter (an Italian deli, if there is one nearby). A good starting point is buffalo mozzarella, torn or sliced, drizzled with olive oil, and sprinkled with salt and some sliced chilli/basil leaves. Add some quality sliced meat such as Parma ham, prosciutto, bresaola and salami and garnish with marinated artichokes, olives, sun-dried tomatoes, roasted bell peppers, capers and gherkins. Add some shavings of Parmesan cheese, and drizzle with some extra virgin olive oil. Meats can be wrapped around grissini (breadsticks) for easy nibbles. Serve with slices of toasted ciabatta for a more substantial first course.

Main course

For the main, something simple is acceptable – but it has to be top-quality simple, perfectly executed and well presented. So, if you are cooking pasta, pay extra for the artisanal Italian spaghetti, and the sauce should go beyond what you would make for yourself on a night in. Basically, go top shelf all the way.

The ideal main is one you can cook while looking nonchalant and holding a conversation – which is why a one-pot meal works well, or anything you can prep in advance and stick in the oven. This risotto ticks all the boxes.

Prawn and asparagus risotto

Risotto needs half an hour of focused cooking, but as long as you have everything else prepared, it's mostly just stirring, allowing you to chat at the same time. Moreover, once you've made a couple of risottos you can call yourself an expert and start to experiment. For instance, in addition to trying out different ingredients in the risotto itself, leftovers can be rolled into balls, dipped in egg and breadcrumbs and fried or baked to make arancini – an excellent portable lunch option.

Serves 2

Ingredients

◆ 200g/7oz raw tiger prawns/shrimp, in their shells
◆ 5cm/2in piece of celery
◆ 1 bay leaf
◆ 50g/2oz/¼ cup butter
◆ 1 small onion, or two echalion (banana) shallots, peeled and finely sliced
◆ 1 bunch thin asparagus, washed, woody bottoms snapped off, and heads removed, stems sliced
◆ 500ml/17fl oz/generous 2 cups good-quality fish stock
◆ 150g/5oz/⅔ cup arborio rice
◆ 1 small glass white wine (and one for the chef)
◆ ½ red chilli, seeded and finely chopped
◆ zest and juice ½ lemon
◆ handful grated Parmesan cheese, plus extra to serve
◆ glug white vermouth
◆ few sprigs of fresh dill (optional), and lemon wedges, to serve

Method

1 Place the prawns/shrimp in a pan, just cover with water, then cook on a medium heat for 4–5 minutes, until they turn pink. Remove from the pan with a slotted spoon, leaving the stock in the pan. When cool enough to handle, peel, setting the prawns aside, and returning the shells to the pan containing the stock.

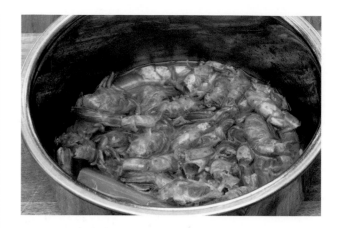

2 Add the celery, if you have it, and a bay leaf, to the prawn stock then boil the liquid until it has reduced to about 100ml/3½fl oz/scant ½ cup.

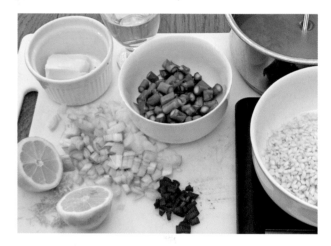

3 Meanwhile, prepare all the other ingredients – once you start cooking the risotto you can't wander off. In a large pan, gently sauté the sliced onion (or shallot) in half the butter for about 15 minutes, until translucent and soft. Make sure they don't brown at all.

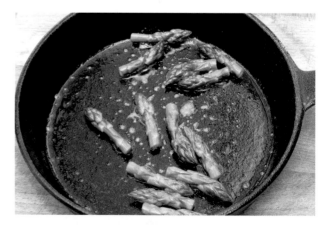

4 Meanwhile, fry the asparagus heads in 5ml/1 tsp of the remaining butter for 1 minute, until tender.

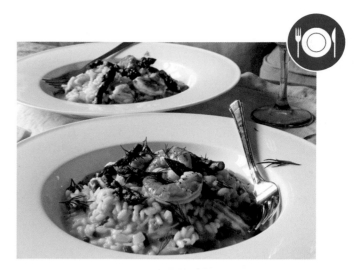

5 Scoop out the prawn/shrimp shells, celery and bay leaf from the reduced liquid, then add the fish stock. Heat to simmering point, then reduce the heat to low.

6 Add the rice to the pan containing the onions and cook, stirring, until the rice is shiny. Pour in the wine and simmer, still stirring, until it has totally evaporated.

7 Start to add the hot stock, a ladleful at a time, stirring continuously. When each ladleful is absorbed, add the next. This will take about 20–30 minutes in total, until the rice is cooked al dente. Halfway through this process, add the sliced asparagus stalks.

10 Ladle the risotto on to warmed plates, top with the asparagus heads, fresh dill, and a little more Parmesan. Serve with lemon wedges for squeezing over.

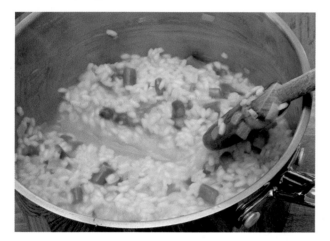

8 When the rice is cooked, the risotto should still be slightly soupy – test by drawing draw the spoon through it and looking for a wake that holds for a few seconds.

Dessert

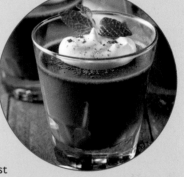

By all means, cheat a little on dessert. If you know where to get the best artisanal ice cream in town, buy it, but maybe add your own twist by sandwiching it between really great cookies or shortbread. It shows the same care and attention to detail as making one yourself, without adding extra pressure. If you do make something, keep it simple and make ahead. Everyone loves chocolate mousse, and it's very easy to make. Serve in little shot glasses or espresso cups and decorate with whipped cream, raspberries or fresh mint for an elegant end to the meal.

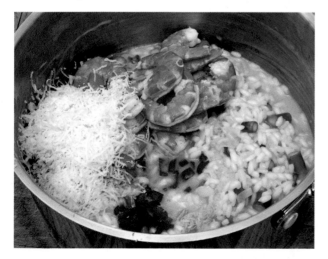

9 Finally, add the prawns/shrimp, chilli, lemon juice and zest, the remaining butter and a handful of Parmesan to the pan. Stir through, on the heat, adding another half-ladle of stock if needed to keep the creamy texture. Stir in a glug of white vermouth and serve straight away.

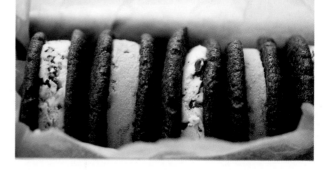

DINNER FOR FOUR

Entertaining is scalable – which means, planned right, it can be no more stress to cook for four (or more) than it is for two. Planning is everything here. You do not want to be the host who abandons guests who barely know each other while you disappear into the kitchen to curse and scream at a fallen soufflé. That means working out in advance what the menu will look like.

You should aim for a balance of tastes and flavours, so think about how the dishes complement and contrast with each other. For instance, a rich appetiser might precede a lighter main, meat might follow seafood, a cold soup could come before a hot entrée. Ensure you have enough plates, cutlery and glasses for everyone coming.

Everything you can do in advance, do. Lay the table, pour the drinks (nominate a friend to be topper-upper, with the responsibility of making sure everyone has a full glass), set out nibbles. For extra points, make some yourself, or customise store-bought ones – it's easy to toast some almonds in the pan with paprika. The line between nibbles and a more formal appetiser can be blurred with a giant platter – eg the Antipasti suggestion on p45.

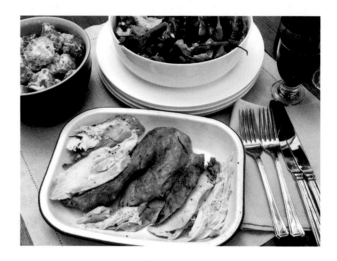

Main course

For the main course, something that can be prepared the previous day is ideal. Moreover, some dishes benefit from having time to sit and mellow, eg chilli. Alternatively, go for an oven-baked dish that can be made in advance (be sure you have enough oven space/roasting pans). For an informal, help-yourself mood, serve it at the table. To get the restaurant effect, plate up in the kitchen – which will allow you to pimp it all up a bit more.

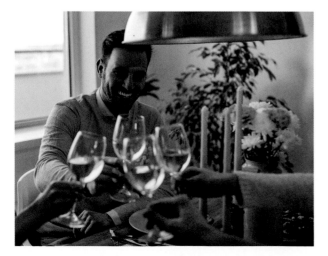

Side dishes

Cold sides, prepared in advance, are ideal. Making a big green salad and ensuring you have plenty of good fresh bread helps to give the impression of a generous meal and adds variety. Serve bread or rolls on a wooden board, alongside a few small shallow bowls of olive oil and balsamic vinegar for dips. If you are serving butter, don't just plonk it on the table: buy posh butter in a cylindrical roll shape and cut it into slim discs. Arrange in a neat row on a dish by the bread so that guests can help themselves. Be sure to lay the table with side plates.

There are also of course thousands of recipes for easy hot side dishes, but a bowlful of colourful steamed seasonal vegetables, perhaps topped with a pat of melting butter, is nearly always appropriate. Frozen peas or broad/fava beans make the perfect stand-by when the fridge is bare. If you're feeling a bit more adventurous, the humble broccoli, cauliflower or kale can easily be elevated to gourmet status by being baked and sprinkled with dukkah, zaatar or seaweed flakes, or blitzed to 'rice' (not the kale) and steamed briefly in a wok with a drop of water to serve as a healthy, low-carb accompaniment. Kale and seaweed crisps are also a tasty, healthy nibble, and easy to make.

HOW TO
ROAST A CHICKEN

If you can roast a chicken, you have access to a wide range of meals and several days of happy eating. Cook this on a Sunday as an excuse to have someone over, serve with roast potatoes and veg, then use leftovers for lunchtime sandwiches, risotto, pie, soup, salad, stir-fries and noodles.

Don't buy factory-farmed chicken unless you really can't afford better; a free-range, higher-welfare bird will have a much better flavour (and a less depressing life), the meat is less likely to dry out during cooking, and the bones make more nutritious stock.

A full roast dinner means a lot of time in the kitchen juggling dishes that need to be ready at the same moment, meaning abandoned guests and a hot, stressed chef. So, if you are cooking this for other people, serve it with dishes you can make ahead, such as potato salad and mixed leaves, or a crispy slaw and crusty bread. You can also serve roast chicken with roasted vegetables (see p31) and couscous or, halfway through cooking, add root vegetables around the chicken for a one-pot meal. Alternatively, make a rice or barley-based risotto, some of which you use to stuff the bird, and the rest you serve as an accompaniment.

Serves 4

Ingredients

- 1.6kg/3½lb free-range chicken
- 1 small onion, peeled
- ½ lemon
- olive oil
- 2 bay leaves and a sprig of rosemary, sage or thyme
- white wine or water (optional)
- salt and ground black pepper
- potato salad and salad leaves, to serve

Method

1 Remove the chicken from the fridge an hour before you start cooking, so that it is at room temperature when it goes in the oven. Preheat the oven to 220°C/425°F/Gas 7.

2 Place the chicken in a roasting tray and push the onion inside the cavity, followed by the half lemon, squeezing it to release the juices as you do so. Push the bay leaves or a sprig of rosemary or sage inside too.

3 Trickle some olive oil over the outside of the chicken and use your hands to rub all over. Season well and place some more rosemary on top.

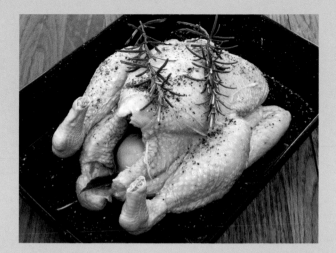

4 Place the chicken in the hot oven. After 15 minutes, turn down the heat to 180°C/350°F/Gas 4 and roast for 1 hour 20 minutes, basting with the juices once or twice. If the pan looks dry, add a splash of white wine or water to the bottom to create some moisture.

5 At the end of the time, the chicken should be cooked – check by inserting a knife into the inside of a leg (the breast cooks first). If no juice runs out it is close to being over-cooked, if a little clear juice runs out it's done to perfection. If juice tinged with pink runs out, it needs another 5–10 minutes.

6 Once cooked, remove from the oven, cover and let the chicken rest for at least half an hour – this relaxes the meat and makes it more tender. Slice and serve with potato salad and salad leaves, or any other accompaniments of your choice.

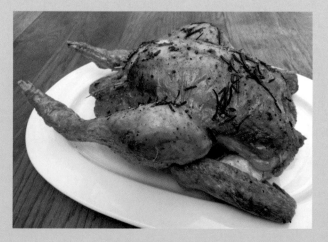

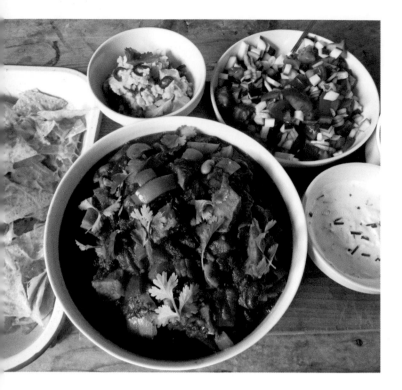

Smoky bean chilli

This recipe is ideal if you have a crowd to feed. Make it a day ahead so all you need to do on the day is rustle up the sides and salsas. Cook rice if you want to, but with warmed tortilla breads and a pile of cheesy nachos it isn't necessary. These quantities serve 6, and will stretch to 8.

Serves 6

Ingredients

- 4 sweet potatoes, peeled and cut into bite-size chunks
- 3 carrots, peeled and cut into chunks
- 30–45ml/2–3 tbsp olive oil
- 5ml/1 tsp each of cayenne pepper, ground cumin, cinnamon and ground coriander
- 3 onions, peeled and roughly chopped
- 3 celery sticks, washed and sliced
- 4 garlic cloves, peeled and minced
- 2 fresh red chillies, finely chopped (seeded if preferred)
- 2 fresh green chillies, finely chopped (seeded if preferred)
- 5ml/1 tsp smoked paprika
- 10ml/2 tsp smoked chipotle paste
- 100ml/3½fl oz/scant ½ cup Mexican beer
- 3 red bell peppers, seeded and roughly chopped
- 2 yellow bell peppers, seeded and roughly chopped
- 1 bunch fresh coriander/cilantro
- 4 × 400g/14oz cans red kidney and pinto beans, drained
- 4 × 400g/14oz cans tomatoes
- juice of half a lemon
- salt and ground black pepper

Method

1 Preheat the oven to 180°C/350°F/Gas 4. Place the diced sweet potatoes and carrots in a large roasting tray, drizzle with olive oil, and mix in the cayenne pepper, cumin, cinnamon and ground coriander. Roast in the oven for 20–30 minutes, until slightly charred. Set aside.

2 Meanwhile, in a very large pan, gently fry the onions and celery for about 15 minutes, stirring from time to time, until soft and slightly golden.

3 Add the garlic and chopped chillies and fry until the aromas are released. Add the smoked paprika and the chipotle paste to the pan and stir through, pour in the beer and use to deglaze the pan (scrape up all the brown bits), then bubble until it has evaporated.

4 Add the rest of the vegetables to the pan, together with the stalks of the fresh coriander/cilantro (the leaves are used later), the beans, tomatoes and a generous amount of salt and black pepper.

5 Cover, bring to a simmer, then reduce the heat and cook for 30–40 minutes, or as long as you have, stirring from time to time, until thickened and reduced.

6 When the chilli is ready, with all the vegetables tender but not falling apart, stir in the roasted sweet potato and carrot, with most of the coriander/cilantro or parsley leaves and the lemon juice. Taste. Add salt and pepper if needed. If you want more heat, add some chilli sauce.

7 Serve hot, garnished with the reserved herbs and your chosen accompaniments.

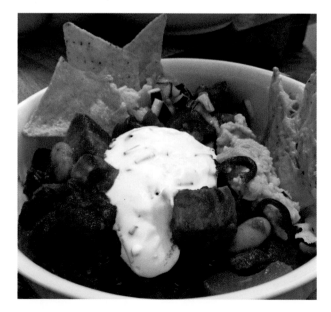

Easy fish pie

This has all the comfort of a classic fish pie without the effort, and can be easily adapted to serve more people. You don't need exact quantities, so mix and match whatever fish is available (white fish or salmon only, not oily or 'blue' fish such as mackerel) and add more crème fraîche and topping as needed.

Serves 4

Ingredients

- 350g/12oz white fish fillets, such as cod, haddock or hake
- 200g/7oz lightly smoked salmon fillets, or un-dyed smoked haddock
- 150g/5oz cooked, peeled prawns/shrimp
- 300ml/½ pint/1¼ cups full-fat crème fraîche
- squeeze of lemon juice
- few sprigs of fresh dill (optional)
- 150g/5oz/generous cup grated extra mature/sharp Cheddar cheese
- handful of panko breadcrumbs
- handful of grated Parmesan cheese
- salt, ground black pepper and paprika
- steamed greens, singed broccoli or salad, to serve

Method

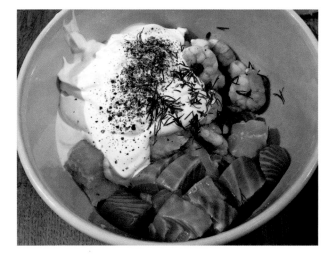

1 Preheat the oven to 180°C/350°F/Gas 4. Cut the fish into large chunks of similar size and place them in a large bowl. Add the prawns/shrimp, crème fraîche, lemon juice, dill, and a good seasoning of salt and ground black pepper. Mix gently until combined.

2 Lightly butter an ovenproof dish and pour in the fish and cream mixture. Top with grated Cheddar. Mix a couple of handfuls of panko breadcrumbs with the same amount of grated Parmesan.

Dessert

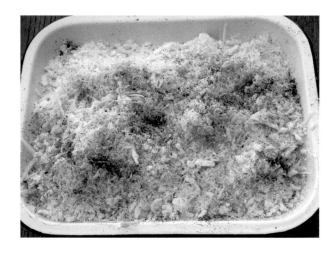

With a larger group you are perfectly entitled to keep it super simple. Cheese is the classic, easy way to end a meal. Two or three large pieces of really good cheese look more elegant than lots of little ones. Arrange on a board with some fruit, nuts, chutneys and crackers and open a good bottle of wine. A dessert wine such as Sauternes or a white Riesling is a good choice to accompany cheese, since the tannins in red tend to drown the creaminess.

3 Sprinkle the breadcrumb mixture over the top. Bake in the oven for about 30 minutes, until the top is crispy and the sauce is bubbling. Serve with greens or salad.

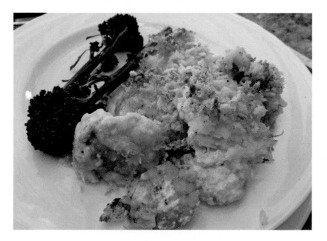

WHAT TO DRINK

Treated with respect, alcohol can lubricate life, bring cheer to social events and empower your visits to the dance floor. If you do choose to drink, teach yourself to savour the good stuff, to recognise good wine and beer, to mix a cocktail for every occasion, and you'll access a world of subtle pleasures.

Appreciating wine

Wine is a drink a man can learn to love deeply, rewarding any effort you put in to studying it. The great fanfare around its appreciation may feel designed to keep it as the pretentious preserve of the special few, but in truth, all you need to savour wine is a nose, a tongue and an imagination. Learning to recognise what you like in a bottle is a useful and rewarding life skill, which will save you from having to dissemble in a restaurant, or randomly pick the second-cheapest option on the list.

It isn't actually necessary to know much more about a wine than whether you like it, and if you're happy to leave it there, your job is simple. Taste it. If it's nice, drink it. Look for that bottle, or that region/varietal, next time. But if you want more – if you want to appreciate the subtle flavours that make one wine great and another just good – learn to concentrate on what you are drinking, and think about how it smells, tastes, feels. At the very minimum, this will allow you to identify when a wine is bad – and when you can send it back.

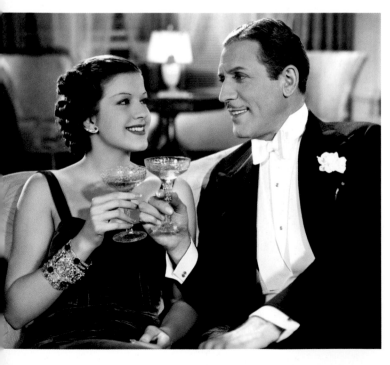

Reading a wine label

Wine labels contain critical information about the stuff in the bottle – and a lot of extraneous detail. To make matters worse, habits and laws are different in different countries. Newer wine countries – eg Australia, America – are more likely to keep it simple and give you the basics, like varietal, upfront and centre. For old-world wines (eg France) you'll need to do some work to understand the information.

Narrowing it down, you are looking for:

- ◆ **Country of origin:** where it was made
- ◆ **Producer:** who made it (usually in big, obvious text)
- ◆ **Year of production:** the vintage. A wine's quality can be hugely impacted by the growing conditions in the year in which it was made. 'NV' stands for Non-Vintage, which means a mix of different years – often used for a consistent taste in familiar brands. TIP: older doesn't mean better. Most of the wines you will encounter in supermarkets are made to be drunk now.
- ◆ **Region:** the area in which the grapes used to make the wine were grown. As a rule of thumb, the bigger the area identified, the cheaper the wine, and vice versa.
- ◆ **Appellation:** the region in which the wine is produced. A wine whose label shows its appellation (eg Champagne, Chablis, etc) will have been produced according to the strict rules of that region.
- ◆ **Alcohol level:** ABV or Alcohol By Volume is expressed as a %. This is not just about how drunk you will get – it has a big impact on taste.

Everything in moderation

As with all good things, it is easy to overdo booze and form bad habits. Keep an eye on yourself. If you find yourself drinking every night, if you are always the guy who wants to keep going when your friends are done, if you are regretting what you did last night – or can't remember what that was – you may have an issue. Talk to someone.

HOW TO
MAKE COCKTAILS

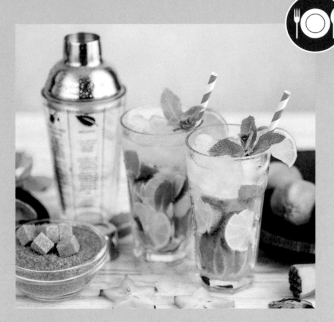

Start by learning how to make a drink that you yourself enjoy. Don't skimp on booze or mixers — cheap tonic ruins a G&T. You can make a lot of good drinks with little more than a glass and some ice cubes, but for impressive cocktails, invest in a shaker and a range of glassware.

There are countless recipes for cocktails online and in books, so look up ones you like and have a go at making them. Build mixology confidence with a couple of classics — the Martini and the Mojito.

Martini
Start with very, very cold gin. Keep a bottle in the freezer — and if you have room, chill the Martini glasses too.

Ingredients
◆ 75ml/2½fl oz gin (an old-fashioned classic — Boodles, Plymouth — works better than a busy 'craft' gin)
◆ 15ml/1 tbsp dry vermouth (the less vermouth you put in, the 'drier' the drink)
◆ cracked ice (if necessary, smash cubes with a rolling pin or similar)
◆ a green olive or a lemon twist, to garnish

Method
1 Pour the gin and vermouth into a shaker filler with cracked ice.
2 Stir for a good while, or shake if you feel Bondish, then strain into the chilled glass.
3 Garnish with one green olive, or a twist of lemon peel.

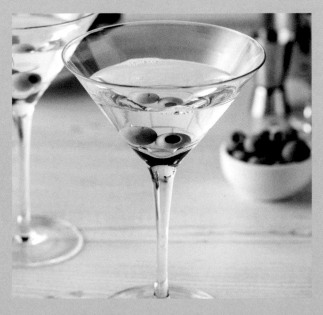

Mojito
Refreshing and tropical, this is a drink for poolside holidays, or times when you want to remember one.

Ingredients
◆ 2 limes, cut into wedges
◆ big handful mint leaves
◆ 10ml/2 tsp sugar
◆ ice
◆ 50ml/2fl oz/¼ cup white rum
◆ soda water

Method
1 Put the limes, mint and sugar into a glass — nothing too fragile. Smash repeatedly with a handy object — the end of a rolling pin will do it. You are releasing the flavour of the mint and the juice from the lime.
2 Throw the ice into the mix and add the rum, giving it a final stir before topping up with soda water. If serving for a guest, add another — un-smashed — mint leaf for decoration.

Mix it up
Regular experimentation should leave you with a good mix of ingredients. At the minimum, for regular cocktail nights you will want to have in a decent bottle of gin, vodka and whisky (save the single malt for sipping neat — blended scotch and a quality bourbon will do for mixing) and rum. Vermouth is a subtle but key ingredient in many great cocktails, and a little bottle of bitters (Angostura is the classic) can make a cocktail sing.

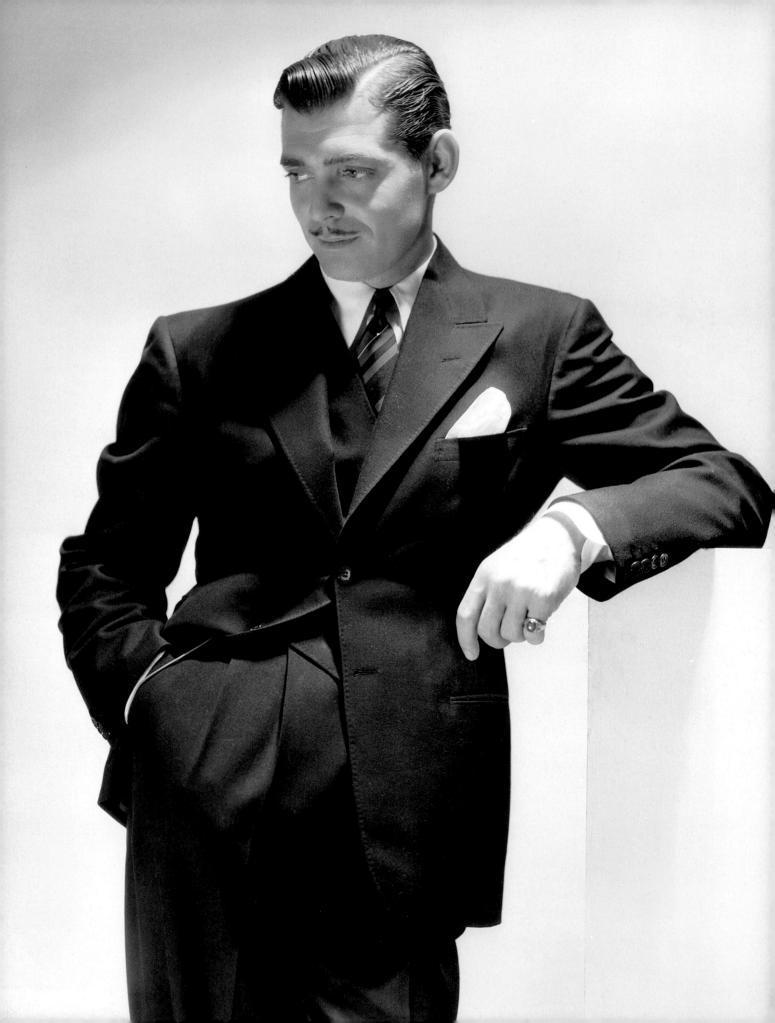

CHAPTER 3
STYLE SECRETS

You are judged, every day, on what you wear; on the fit of your trousers and the state of your shoes. It affects your career, your relationships, and your self-esteem; it's worth spending both time and effort on. The pages that follow offer guidance on making the most of what you've got and focuses not on fashion (which changes all the time) but style, which is permanent.

FINDING YOUR STYLE

Style isn't following trends, or obeying a set of rules. To rock a look that makes the best of what you have, you must own it. If you choose an outfit because it's what you've been told to wear there is a risk that you will come across as uncomfortable. A man should assemble a collection of clothes that project his inner life to the outside world and reflect his personality.

Purge

Before you assemble a new look, audit your existing wardrobe. Be brutal. Lay out all your clothing, including gym gear etc. Try it all on, piece by piece, shoes too. Check the fit, check how you look in the mirror. Ask yourself if you love it, if it makes you look good, or if you've worn it in the last year. If it's a 'no', chuck it. Learn lessons from what you throw out, and what you are keeping.

Building your style

If you are going to reinvent or refresh your style, it helps to have a sense of direction. Start paying closer attention to how other men dress. Whose style do you admire? Someone in the office, a friend, a TV presenter? Look closely at the details of what they are wearing – why does it work, could it work for you? Inspiration is available all around – on the street or Internet, in style mags, TV programmes, old movies. In this chapter we've included some icons, but there is a lot to be said for finding your own role models. This is not about stealing or replicating what someone else wears, but learning from it, and finessing your approach.

▼ Assemble a wardrobe around what works for you.

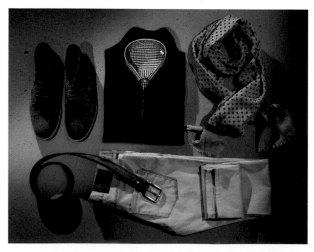

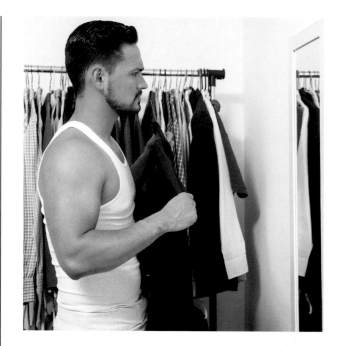

Think too about how you live. Work/home/lifestyle doesn't have to define you, and if you've got the nerve there is a lot to be said for rocking a style that sticks two fingers up to the norms. However, if you live on a dairy farm, a white suit and Italian loafers are never going to be suitable.

Allow yourself the freedom to think big, and consider totally reinventing your style. You're conceiving an idea of the ideal you, and it costs nothing to use your imagination.

'I can go all over the world with just three outfits: a blue blazer and grey flannel pants, a grey flannel suit, and black tie'
Pierre Cardin

Building a collection

You're looking to collate and curate a wardrobe of clothes that work together – so it helps to have a framework, to narrow things down. Work out which colours suit you and which don't, and claim this as a palette you can stick to. It will help ensure what you buy works with the rest of your wardrobe. Set a core colour scheme for the basics – and be more adventurous on the accessories.

Compile a list of no-no's in terms of colour, fit, style. This should include a ban on anything that pinches or is uncomfortable to wear. Buy clothes for who you are now, not who you hope to be after a crash diet or a gym habit.

Rock what you've got…

Every man has something going for him. A feature that is his alone and that, brought to the fore, will make him look his best. Your job is to find it, and let it work for you.

Your efforts should be concentrated on promoting your advantages and building on your strengths. If you can't identify them, ask someone you can trust (and have a word with yourself about self-esteem). It could be your eyes, height, physique, or something more intangible – swagger, charm, cheek. Work with those features – if you've got bright-blue eyes, wear a shirt in a similar shade. If you're proud of a toned torso, wear your tops on the slimmer side. If your USP is more to do with your personality, think about how you dress now expresses or conceals who you are.

Some things about the way you look can be changed, and some cannot. Waistlines can be adjusted, with effort, and problem hair can be cut and styled. Height is more difficult, and most 'cures' for baldness don't work.

It is natural to focus on the things you don't like about your looks – but if that's all you see when you look in the mirror, it will show. The only thought worth giving to your shortcomings is how you might minimise them. So, a shorter man may want a suit that elongates and hair that lifts the eye up rather than down, whereas a bigger man may want clothes that help create a slimming silhouette. The man with thinning hair may want to make the most of what he has – but at a certain point there is a lot to be said for shaving it off and putting your effort into your style instead.

The pressure to conform

Many guys feel a pressure to conform to a certain look, based in part on highly selective and carefully edited images chucked at them via social media and advertising. Some may push themselves and their bodies towards their idea of a masculine ideal. However, there are many body types, and while there's nothing wrong with making the most of what you have, bear in mind that not everyone

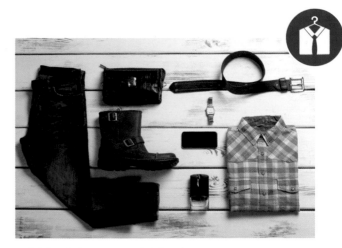

▲ Only buy clothes you love, which fit and suit you.

was made to be ultra-bulky, or whippet thin. Accepting and embracing your own build and working with it, with clothes that suit and fit, is a quicker path to looking good than what you will get from protein shakes and a gym addiction.

Many men are expected to conform to a certain style of dress, at least in the workplace or for formal occasions – but as the forward-thinking gentleman has always known, there is great pleasure to be had from ignoring the rules and letting your freak flag fly a bit. Life is short – if you want to wear a pink suit to a wedding but think your friends might take the piss, wear the suit and laugh along – or make some new friends.

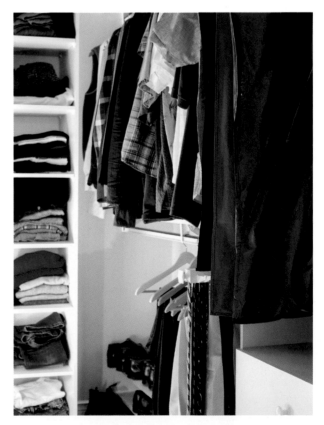

TOP MEN

In a world full of difficult decisions and too many options, it helps to have a role model. The men in the pages that follow have been cited as the best-dressed fellows of the modern era. They set the template that fashion designers and stylists draw from/rip off – looks that flatter most men, which feel ageless and outside of the whims of fashion. You don't have to copy these details slavishly – though if you did, odds are you'd look pretty damn good.

Steve McQueen

Steve McQueen was one of the best-dressed men of his era – the King of Cool, a Hollywood star who women loved and men wanted to be. What worked for him 50 years ago can work for you now.

It's all in the attitude – and the attention to detail. The look is simple, but deadly effective – McQueen has taken the time to think about every individual piece of clothing, and pulled together a perfectly coordinated style without looking vain or self-interested. The effort is there, but hidden, and the vibe reflects his motto: 'I live for myself and I answer to nobody.' Everything fits – and flatters his physique.

A costume designer told me she once watched McQueen try on 30 pairs of almost identical trousers before he found the ones he felt suited him. You can learn from this: be exacting with your style, and never settle for anything less than perfect.

Lessons

- A stylish old-school watch works with nearly everything (though not ideal if you're running a marathon…) – it's the one piece of jewellery a man can flash without looking too try-hard.
- Buy classic items and you will never be out of style.
- Only ever buy clothes you love, which suit you and fit you. If it isn't perfect, don't bother.
- Aim high, but be yourself.

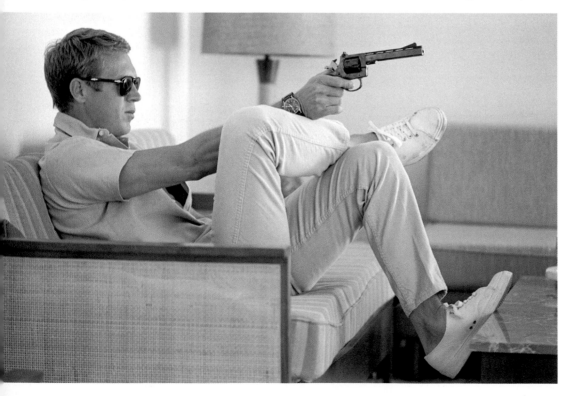

◀ McQueen is wearing a slim-fit short-sleeved shirt with a button-down collar, white Levi's and classic Jack Purcell Converse. The simplicity of his style draws attention to the well-chosen accessories – the Persol 714 sunglasses, the functional but elegant watch (a rare Hanhart 417). You can still buy every one of those items, bar the watch, so it's possible to borrow the look wholesale – though to avoid smelly feet you might want to invest in low-rise cotton ankle socks…

JAMES BOND

Spoiler alert: James Bond isn't real. Nevertheless, he is many people's idea of the best-dressed man of this and any other age. In the books, Fleming specifies every aspect of Bond's tastes, from his cigarettes to his car to his tailor – an attention to detail that was carried through to the films. The look was classic, but contemporaneous – always in step with the style of the era, but not so much that you would point at it and laugh 10 years later.

In suits, Bond personified the British gentleman – without necessarily wearing British tailoring. His was a formal look, correct according to the rules of style (Bond knew a man was a wrong 'un by the fashion laws he broke) but modern, with just a hint of flash. It was also attitude: supremely confident and at home in his outfits – a quiet swagger that carries through his formal wear and his off-duty wardrobe. In keeping with Fleming's scrupulous approach, every single item is carefully chosen. More than that – it is appropriate for the job at hand. Bond is not running around a North African souk in tweed – he's in desert boots and a short-sleeved shirt.

Lessons

◆ Only wear items you love. Buying the best you can afford is a good place to start.
◆ Project confidence. Know you look good and others will too. NB confidence is not arrogance, and arrogance is not attractive.
◆ Know the rules. Even if you're going to break them.
◆ Dress for where you are and who you are. Don't put one above the other.
◆ Buy a good suit.
◆ Keep it simple. If you are dressed to the nines, check yourself in the mirror before leaving the house, and consider removing one item.

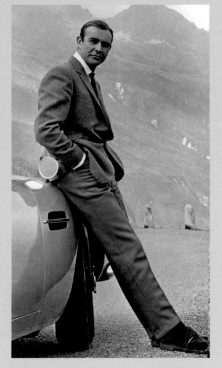

⌃ Sean Connery exuding confidence in his 'Sunday motoring' threads.

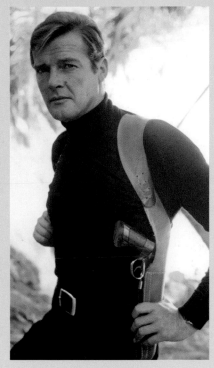

⌃ Roger Moore discards the suit for an outfit that is suitable for action, but also shows that style doesn't date.

▽ Pierce Brosnan strikes the classic Bond pose while wearing the black tie ensemble for which the character is most famous.

▽ Daniel Craig has taken Bond into the 21st century, his look is sharp, precise, expensive and fit.

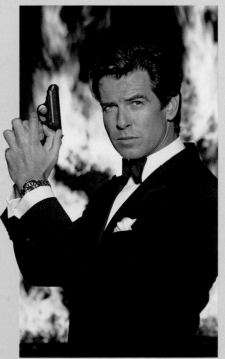

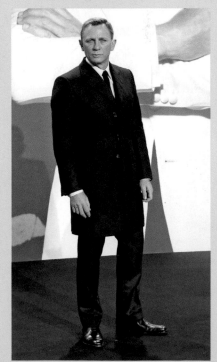

Marcello

There's a word for Marcello Mastroianni, and it sums up the ideal approach to men's style: *sprezzatura*. It's a word that could only exist in Italian – meaning the art of achieving something difficult while looking like you haven't even tried. This is the magic of Marcello. He never looks less than great, but equally doesn't look like he particularly cares. He is generally in a suit, usually an elegant, unfussy two-button single-breasted one, with a crisp white shirt and contrasting tie. The secret of his success is in the quality of the suit – the cut, the material and the fit.

Lessons

◆ Choose your clothes carefully – and then stop worrying about them.
◆ Cool means not having to try. Keep any effort invisible.
◆ Have the confidence to take a small risk now and again – personalise what you wear.
◆ Quality, simple clothes can be devastatingly effective.

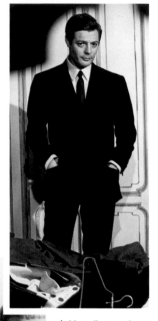

∧ Marcello, utterly at home in a suit and tie.

‹ Not every man can rock a white suit.

Tom Hardy

When he goes for it, Hardy wears the hell out of a suit, and it is clear from his bearing that he knows it. The contrast between the face-fuzz/ink/beefy physique and the sharp, defined tailoring is pure chemistry and the short-back-and-sides haircut gives him the feel of an old-school ruffian. This is not a man who looks like he has borrowed his uncle's suit for a job interview. He looks like he has styled himself and pleased himself – and if you don't like it, that's your problem.

Lessons

◆ Please yourself. Own it.
◆ Accessorise with imagination.
◆ Keep it simple.
◆ Manly contrasts nicely with sharp/smart clothes. Try not shaving but wearing a tie.
◆ A sturdy guy looks good in sturdy gear.

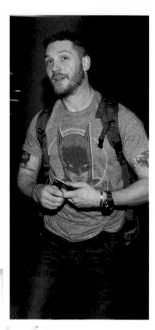

∧ In civvies, Hardy exudes nonchalant confidence.

‹ The man wears a suit like he owns it.

Pharrell Williams

The main lesson to take away from Pharell's look is that you are not Pharrell. What he does, and how he does it, would not work with anyone else. He understands the rules of men's style, and ignores them. And that's the trick – his USP is that he is his own man (that, and the buffalo hat). He loves clothes, loves playing around with them. This could come across as incoherent madness, but instead it works as wild genius – there is always a careful thought behind the look, and a vibe on which he is riffing. This guy's style tells us to lighten up, to wear whatever we damn well please and be happy about it.

Lessons

◆ Contrast is good. Mix it up, but think it through.
◆ Be your own brand.
◆ Feel free to customise clothes to your own ideas.
◆ Take a risk with colour. Most men don't, so those who do stand out.

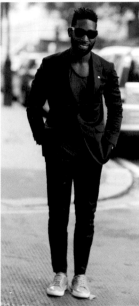

︿ Pharrell knows the rules, and breaks them.

‹ A man of style isn't afraid of colour…

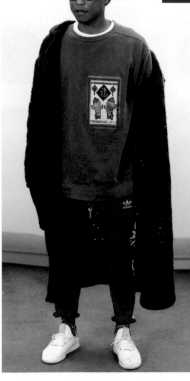

Tinie Tempah

Tinie calls his approach to style 'street cool'. His understanding of new trends is informed by a deep knowledge of formal menswear and of the real purpose of style – to make a man look good. Being up to date never means sacrificing a flattering silhouette, or playing against your strengths. There's an element of risk, of pushing boundaries and breaking rules, but it is carefully calculated. Trousers are worn an inch too short – but with the sockless loafer it becomes the trademark of a personal style.

Lessons

◆ Style is not just what you wear, but how you wear it.
◆ Have a consistent element that is a key part of your look – and own it.
◆ If you're going to break the rules, it helps to know what they are.
◆ Keep it fresh – try new things, new looks.

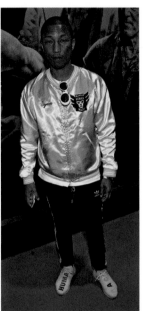

︿ Tinie showing how a suit can work for everyday wear.

‹ Box-fresh classic trainers can work with a suit.

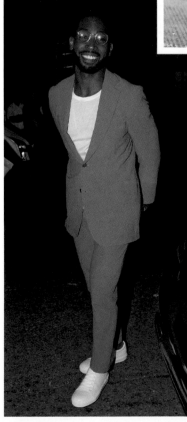

THE STAPLES

Assembling a great wardrobe does not mean stuffing a cupboard with an assortment of fabulous clothes. It means thinking each purchase through carefully, aiming for consistency and a collection that works in various combinations and various settings. It also means buying fewer but better items. Keeping it simple and classic will give you less to do in the long run.

Fashion vs style

Chasing fashion and striving to remain up to date is a lifestyle that works for some men. If that's you, by all means go for it. If not, there is little to be gained from trying to keep up with catwalk trends, except in the loosest sense. If your interest is in looking good, focus on style, not fashion. One is about looking contemporary. One is about looking good.

What we've suggested here is a core collection, with a heavy emphasis on classic, grown-up style that will work for most men. Take this advice with a pinch of salt and add or subtract based on your personal style and interests … clearly, if you are a goth you won't be wanting bright polo shirts, chinos or loafers.

Slim chinos

The chino is a great utilitarian trouser for the modern man and an alternative to jeans – smart enough to pass muster on a date or for work, casual enough for weekend slouch-around wear. Chinos are easy to wash and mostly you will not want to bother ironing a crease in. Avoid unflattering pleats – you want a flat-fronted trouser. The fit, especially for a younger guy, should be slim – the magic point between tight (no room for movement) and loose (will never be smart, looks ridiculous with smarter shoes). Chinos can work with or without turn-ups – how high to turn them up is your call, but avoid flashing a section of hairy leg. Any shade on the tan scale between off-white and khaki will do, but blue and grey are similarly flexible.

Spend your money on a few high quality items of clothing that you can dress up and down. A white t-shirt and boots with the same jacket and trousers gives a completely different look to a shirt and tie. If you're used to dressing down, try turning it up a notch by adding a pocket square, or even a waistcoat and cufflinks. You may be surprised at the positive reactions you get.

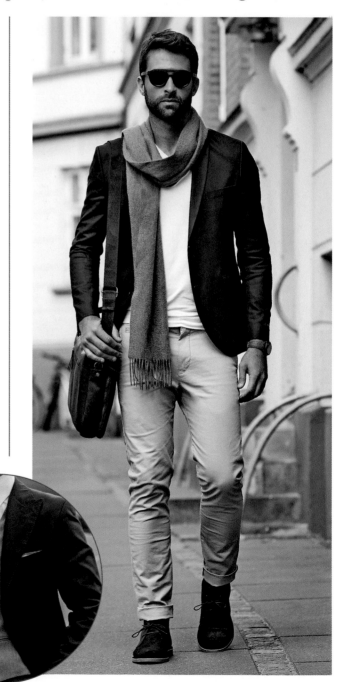

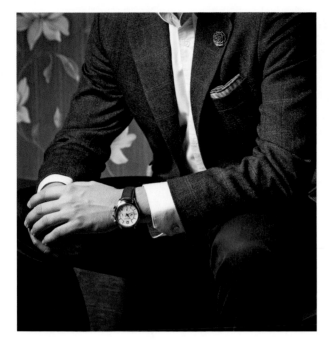

▲ The right pair of well fitting jeans can be dressed up for evening wear with ease. You don't have to wear a tie, just a shirt and a fitted jacket will do.

Dark jeans

A neat pair of well-fitting indigo dark jeans, in good denim, is adaptable to a huge array of outfits/occasions. There are strong arguments for other jeans, but their range is more limited. Smart, slim dark-blue jeans can be dressed up with suede shoes and a jacket, or dressed down with trainers/sneakers and a sweatshirt.

Fit is everything. Take your time, and try on as many pairs as necessary. Remember there is a risk of shrinkage – check the label. The better/heavier the denim, the better it will age. Legs can be shortened – fat turn-ups look good on vintage, casual jeans but can be awkward in combination with a smarter look. For a sharper look, a finished hem is preferable. At the time of writing, spray-on jeans that hug the calf are common and work for some men. However, be aware that 'slim' is generally more flattering than ultra-tight.

Smart grey trousers

Grey is a magic (non) colour – it goes with everything. A smart, well-fitting pair of grey slacks will form the basis for a smart casual work outfit when paired with a shirt and sweater, but really starts to pay its way in combination with a blazer/smart jacket – as smart as a suit, but more interesting to look at.

Suit(s)

Every man needs one suit, and many men need several. See the next chapter for how to buy one that works for you, and will last.

The blazer

If there is one item that will make a well-dressed man of you it is the blazer/sports coat/smart jacket, which works in an incredible variety of contexts. Basically the top half of a suit, but designed to be worn without matching trousers, it looks great with jeans and chinos, or dressed up with a pair of smarter trousers in a contrasting colour. Wear it with a tie or a polo shirt or a polo neck – and if you insist, with a T-shirt, though that's an easy look to get wrong. It fits the gap between relaxed and formal, when you want to show you've put some effort in but don't want to go full suit. Buy a solid colour that works with your shirts/trousers, and that is a perfect fit. Single-breasted is more flexible than double.

▶ Button-down shirts can be worn with or without a tie.

▼ Add a cashmere jumper and pocket square for a more smart than casual look.

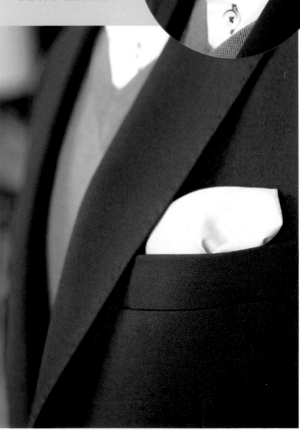

Shorts

If you live somewhere warm enough, or have a holiday planned, incorporate a few pairs of smart shorts into your wardrobe. Chino-style, denim, red-and-white checked gingham, narrow blue/white striped 'seersucker', madras/plaid are all good options. If you are wearing with a simple top – eg a plain white button-down top, or a neutral polo, you can afford to go a little crazy with colour. Shorts that end above the knee are smarter and more flattering than those that dangle below it.

Button-down shirts

A decent button-down shirt is equally at home in an office, bar, or yachting scenario. It has an informality that a more serious work shirt doesn't and so does excellent double duty with chinos or jeans. Crisp white is a good place to start, setting off any skin tone (and especially a tan) but don't eschew light blue – men with blue eyes in particular could potentially embrace this as a trademark look. Good with a tie (square-ended, knitted, particularly), good without. Keep it in a slim cut – avoid puffy folds of cloth mushrooming out above the belt line.

Polo top

The three-button short-sleeve polo top is ubiquitous in most men's wardrobes, and has barely gone out of style over 60 years, for good reason. It gets you a collar, which makes it a more natural partner to a jacket or blazer than a plain T-shirt. Worn in a slim fit, as it should be, it highlights a slender or toned physique particularly well – and worn untucked over jeans/shorts, can help conceal any tummy overspill. Go wild with colour if that's your thing, or keep it neutral. There's no hard rule on collar up – only that you be aware that worn up it can look a little cocky/adolescent or preppy.

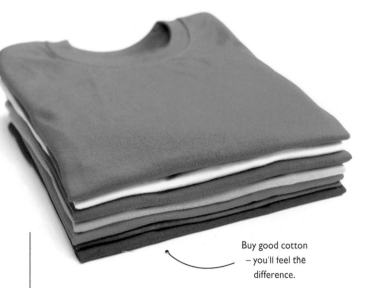

Buy good cotton – you'll feel the difference.

Plain T-shirt

The plain T-shirt serves a variety of purposes. For the man who is proud of his gym time or beach tan, there is no more effective way to offset it. The humble white T also works as an extra layer under shirts, keeping you warmer and protecting your shirts from your armpits. Buy in solid colours that complement your outfits, and invest in good cotton. For more variety and a yachty/Scandi feel, try thick blue-and-white stripes.

Knitwear

Wool – and shoes – are where to spend your money. Buy quality material – it is lighter, warmer and sexier. Everyone wants to touch a man in cashmere, and merino is an affordable second best. Start with a V-neck or cardigan – worn with a suit, these give the impression of a three-piece without the expense and a relaxed look when you remove your jacket. A black polo neck is slimming and flattering, working with almost any combo and lending you an instant artsy vibe. A chunky-knit cardigan with a shawl collar is a stylish option for casual weekend wear.

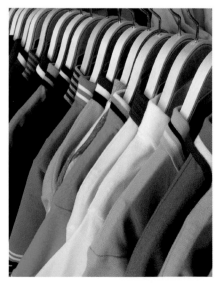

◀ A polo top is a great way to introduce bold colour into your style.

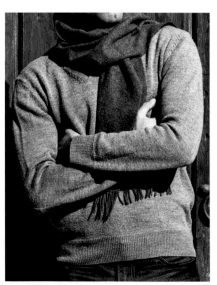

◀ Soft wool looks and feels luxurious.

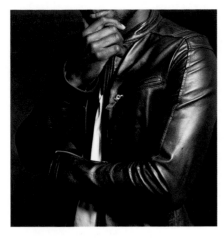

◀ A good leather jacket should fit like a glove, and last you years.

Outerwear

Dressing for inclement weather offers a test of your style credentials. Your comfort is not worth dressing badly for, but being cold and damp is too high a price to pay for looking good. Split the difference, and buy outerwear that does the job in style. A classic trench-coat/mac keeps you dry and looks equally good with a suit and with jeans. A Harrington bomber jacket is a crisp but casual way to top off jeans – unless you feel comfortable rocking the tricky double-denim look, reserve a denim jacket for chinos. Vintage jackets offer instant masculine style – aim for Marlon Brando rather than Jeremy Clarkson. For really foul weather, a man needs a Parka – basically a sleeping bag with arms – while a Scandi-style anorak will repel the worst torrential rain. If you are treating yourself to one outerwear item, make it a good wool overcoat – Crombies are the crème de la crème – a narrow, slim-fitting coat with a velvet collar, ultra-sharp whether dressed up or dressed down.

◀ Every man feels like the don in a Crombie.

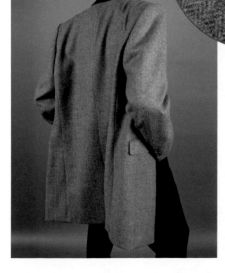

Accessories

If you restrained your colour and pattern choices for the basics, you can afford to take more chances on accessories, choosing ones that express you and work with each other. Go to town on scarves, ties, hats, belts, pocket squares (a hanky for your suit pocket) and socks. A little bit of flair can go a long way.

Don't let down a great look with a terrible bag – this is as much a part of your outfit as your tie. A vintage leather holdall or satchel is an inexpensive and flexible alternative to a briefcase. A backpack is practical; choose one that is of an appropriate size and ergonomically designed so it doesn't hurt your back, and looks good.

A man can never own too many socks. Buy yours with your ties in mind, if you wear them – if not, something that goes with your shirts. Having a variety to play with means you can change up a look easily. With a formal suit or a dress-down ensemble, the sock gives you the opportunity to express a little of yourself – with colours and patterns that echo any other part of your outfit.

▼ Taking care over the little things – a carefully chosen leather belt that matches your shoes, a stylish well-tied tie, a classic watch – will mean you always look good.

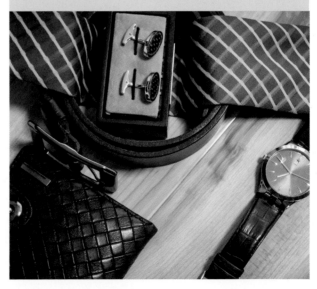

MEN'S SHOES

Oxfords

An Oxford is the classic British man's formal shoe – made for business, sleek and usually black, with 'closed lacing' – the two sides containing the eyelets for the laces join together at the bottom, so laces appear more discreetly tucked away. Best with a suit, and may not work with anything more casual.

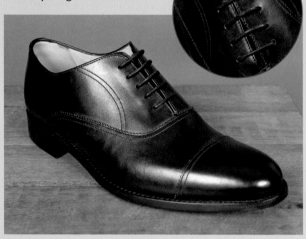

Loafers

If the brogue is the best of British, the loafer is the continental equivalent – light, soft, supple, a slip-on instead of a lace, with some element of frou-frou (a penny, a tassel) for detail. The best are American or Italian. They expose more ankle/sock, so choose your hosiery wisely, or go sockless.

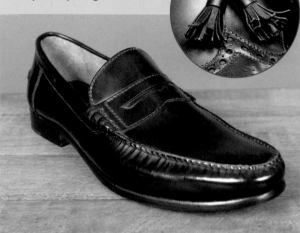

Derbies/'brogues'

Derby shoes are 'open laced' at the bottom, making them slightly wider and more comfortable to put on – and therefore less formal. Strictly speaking, 'brogue' refers only to the punch-hole detailing but in practice the word is shorthand for a traditional, chunky British shoe, of the kind often worn with a more relaxed, tweedy suit, or with jeans/chinos. Because they work with so many outfits and last forever, they are a good investment.

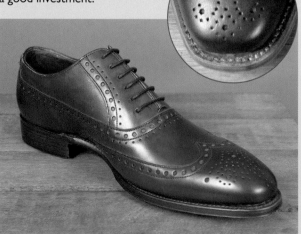

Desert boots

Another very British item, the desert boot was inspired by the off-duty footwear of British Army officers in Africa, and claimed as a style item by the modernists of late 1950s London. Desert boots have crêpe soles, making them light but not particularly hard-wearing – look after them. It's possible to get away with pairing them with a relaxed suit – but they are more at home with a chino or jean.

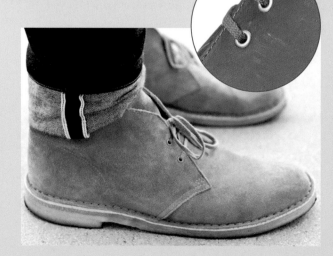

Trainers/sneakers

For classic and flexible, you can't beat a pair of Jack Purcell Converse. A timeless design, now available in a million variations but always best in old-fashioned cream/off-white canvas, they go with anything – if you've got the nerve and they are box fresh you can pair with a casual suit, otherwise denim and khaki are their natural bedfellows. For summer they are a good fit with shorts – try sockless (or invisible short socks). Happily, everything has been reissued, and you can rock an old-school vibe with any casual outfit.

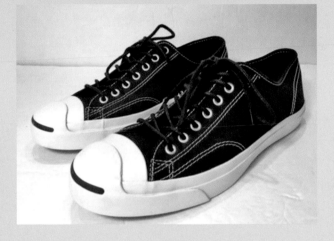

Buying shoes

Buying super-cheap shoes is generally a false economy. A good, well-made pair of leather shoes will give you years of wear, with a bit of care, while ones with plastic soles may not last. You don't need to own all these shoes – though the more you rotate your footwear, the longer it will survive. Most guys will need at least one pair of 'smart' shoes at some point – if money is tight, go for something hard-wearing which can do duty for work and play.

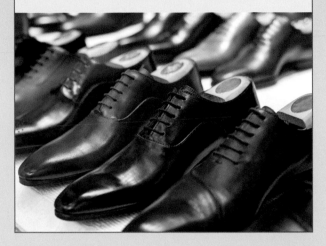

Chelsea boots

When you want a slim silhouette but don't want to show off a bit of sock, Chelsea boots are the answer. Sturdy, but elegant enough to wear with a suit – provided you buy a well-made, well-shaped pair with a low heel, a leather sole and a toe that is neither too pointed (the winkle-picker works best for goths and rockers, and less well in the office) nor round. A chisel toe is the best of both worlds. Black leather boots look good with a grey or navy suit but are harder to wear with jeans – while the reverse is true of brown suede.

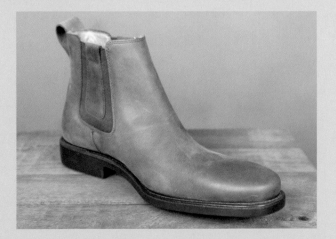

Work boots

Winter can be tough. Be ready with a sturdy pair of US-style work boots, which can do duty for outdoor activities, hiking, Sunday pub walks, travelling in rough terrain or just mooching around town in inclement weather. The chunkier the boot, the less well it will pair with very skinny jeans – works best with a slightly more relaxed fit on the calf.

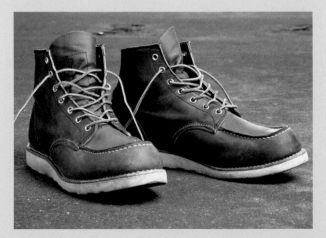

SUITED AND BOOTED

A man in a suit is a man at his best. Despite huge changes in the workplace, the growth of casual sportswear, and the rise of Internet billionaires in grubby T-shirts, a suit remains the ultimate sartorial symbol of power. A matching jacket and trousers are the uniform that says a man is in control of himself and his world, that he commands some authority, sophistication and taste. A well-cut suit flatters a man's physique, hides his flaws and makes him stand taller.

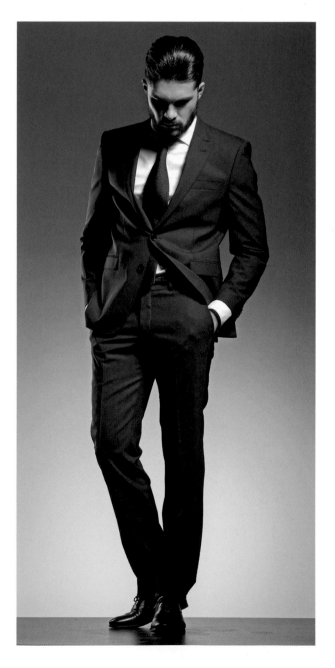

However. Take a look around the average office, the average wedding. How many guys look sharp, confident – and how many look as if they've been forced in to a suit-shaped outfit that will just about do the job?

It doesn't have to be that way. Embrace the suit. There is no better way to dress like a man. Here's how.

Buying a suit

How do you know a suit is for you? The same way you know whom to marry. You know. And if you don't know – if you think, 'Well, maybe, I guess so, it'll do, it's affordable…' then take the suit off and walk away. 'Good enough' means nowhere near good enough, in questions of both love and style. Aim higher.

The three kinds of suit

- ◆ Off-the-rack: Standard-sized suit, bought ready made, but may be altered by the shop or by your tailor. Men who are a 'standard' size (per the rules of fashion) will have more luck in the racks. £
- ◆ Made-to-measure: A suit that is cut for you from a previous pattern (by machine) and adjusted to your measurements. Probably requires one fitting to take your details and a final fitting for any tweaks. If you have trouble finding a ready-made suit that fits, this may be your best bet. ££
- ◆ Bespoke: Created entirely for you, oh lucky man. The best. Multiple fittings and a pattern brought into being by talented craftspeople – just so you can look very, very good. £££££ (but worth it).

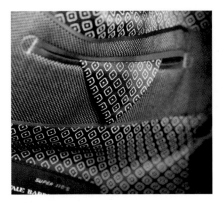

▲ The best suits have a silk lining.

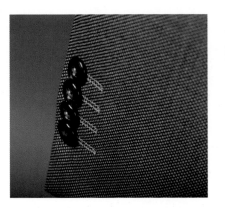

▲ Quality shows in small details, like stitching.

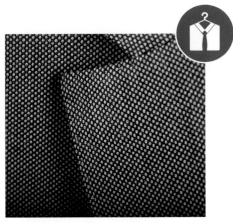

▲ A fine micro-pattern is easier to wear than a loud stripe/check.

More for your money

Put the care into buying a suit that you would put into buying any major item. Start with a budget – what's the most you can afford? Where can you get the most for your money? Maximise your budget by buying in the sales, at discount places – but not online. You need to try this on. There are very cheap suit-shaped objects available in high-street stores, some of which will more or less do the job, but odds are they will not be made to last. Set the bar high, even for a back-up suit. You want quality in the whole squad, not just the first team.

Buying the best you can afford doesn't mean paying full whack for the flashiest designer label. Look instead for the details that are worth your coin: the weight of the material, the quality of the stitching, how it feels to wear. Cheaper suits may be 'fused' – the lining is glued to the outer fabric and may 'bubble' when dry-cleaned, as the fabric comes away from the garment. Polyester linings are common in a cheap suit. This is an uncomfortable fabric, likely to make you sweat. Unless you are in showbusiness, avoid shiny suits, even expensive ones – they rarely look good.

With practice you can learn to recognise quality. Where was it made? The inside label will tell you. Bonus points for places where labour is more expensive and there is a tradition of menswear expertise – Italy, England. Natural fibres (wool, cotton, worsted, silk, cashmere, or any blend thereof) cost more. Anything made from more than a touch of polyester is to be avoided. Scrunch the fabric in your hand – does it feel soft? Does it retain a crease? You will want a heavier cloth for winter warmth and something lighter for summer use. No suit was made to be worn every day. Allow yours a break by owning more than one and rotating or, if the shop sells the trousers as separates, invest in a second pair. They take way more punishment than jackets.

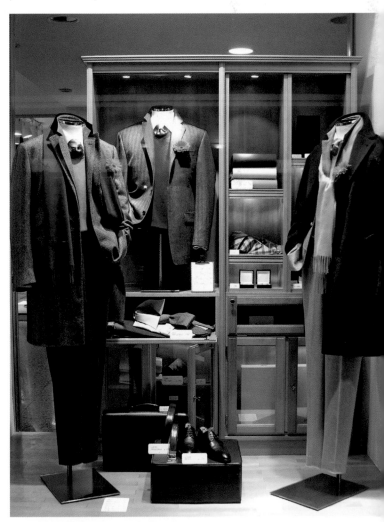

'Clothes don't make a man, but clothes have got many a man a good job'

Herbert Vreeland

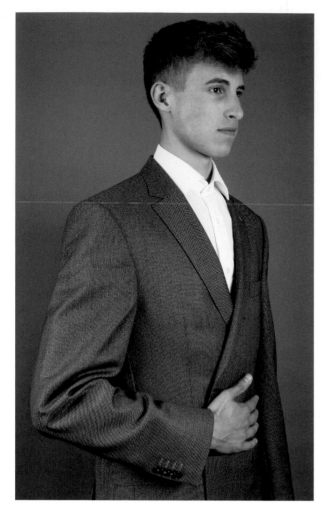

▲ Take all the time you need choosing a suit.

Narrowing it down

Start with questions. What is it for? How often are you going to be wearing this, and where? Is it an everyday option for the office, sober enough to not frighten the client/boss, or for a particular event? Assuming you want this to be *the* suit you will want it to do duty in all of those functions, which helps whittle down your choices considerably.

Unless you work in a world where any kind of suit goes, the odds are you will want to go reasonably conservative. At the time of writing, that probably means a slim single-breasted one with two or three buttons, in a solid colour. It isn't possible to go wrong with a navy blue or charcoal grey single-breasted – the safest, most versatile and flattering options, limiting any confusion over tie/shirt combinations.

That said, there's nothing inherently wrong with a check or a stripe, and it can add interest and variety to your look – but one more thing to think about is one more thing to get wrong. For an easy life, leave the patterns to your accessories, or use a discreet micro-pattern.

Never, ever, do up the bottom button of a single-breasted suit. On a three-button jacket the rule is middle yes, top sometimes, bottom never.

Double-breasted is a dashing look, flamboyant, smart and flattering for some body types, making the upper half of the torso bigger and slimming the waist. Fit is crucial – you don't want a load of excess material flapping about. Suit lapels may be peaked, subtly making more of your manly chest.

Modern double-breasted suits are cut on the slim side – beware going too tight, lest you look like a sausage about to pop its skin. Follow the fit rules given on px, but allow a little more length for the jacket, to compensate for all the activity higher up. A jacket with six buttons is the benchmark, though both eight and four are possible for forward thinkers. Button it up, bar the bottom one.

Trying it on

We've assumed here you are buying off the rack (if you have the money for M-T-M or bespoke, go for it). Trying on a ready-made suit means picking your targets – which shops you are going to hit (check online, in style mags and the outfits of men you admire) and preparing accordingly. Wear smart shoes and a plain shirt. Bring a friend, if you don't trust your judgement. Get measured in the shop, and write down the measurements for future reference. Look down the racks for something that speaks to you – if you narrowed it down to cut/colour already that will help. Try as many on as possible – it's a free education.

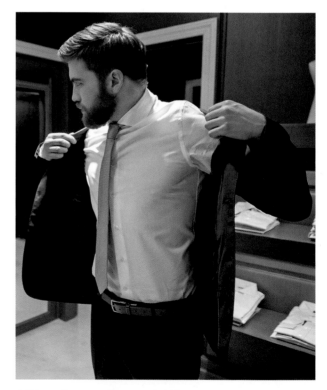

▲ Bring a wing-person for a second opinion.

A SUIT FOR EVERY SIZE

Men's fashion is generally marketed at a 'standard size' guy – when the truth is that mankind comes in a wide variety of shapes and sizes. If you aren't Mr Average (perversely, most guys aren't) don't give up on looking smart – use a careful strategy to play to your strengths.

Smaller men

◆ Go for a slim fit. Baggy, loose clothing makes you shrink visually. Feel free to show a little sock, and wear your trousers slightly higher on the hip to elongate the legs.

◆ Get everything altered to create a perfect fit. Suit and shirt should be carefully matched to your shape, so the wandering eye takes you in as one complete, precise package.

◆ A two-button single-breasted suit creates a V shape that makes the most of your torso. A matching suit brings unity, whereas wearing contrasts splits you up.

◆ Keep it simple. Avoid lots of garish colours. A fine stripe or corduroy will help bring the eye up, elongating you. If you wear a pattern, keep it small and fine.

Taller men

◆ A slim fit is the way to go, but avoid a skinny, spray-on suit – one that's too tight will make you look like a runner bean.

◆ A single-breasted two-button affair, on which the lapels sit slightly higher, helps add width to your shoulders, especially with peaked lapels.

◆ A double-breasted suit is also very good at adding width.

◆ Break it up – wear contrasting jackets and trousers rather than a suit to help define your various regions.

◆ Patterns can give you width and visual interest – try checks.

Big guys

◆ Big men should not be afraid to wear a suit, and definitely shouldn't hide in something shaped like a potato sack. Bigger clothes make you look ill defined and sloppy. Get something that fits.

◆ Look for the cut to help define your shape for the better. Let it hang right at the shoulder, but get it pinched in a touch at the waist – enough to give you a strong silhouette.

◆ Off-the-rack clothing rarely fits the bigger man perfectly – find an alterations tailor and get it tweaked to you.

◆ A single-breasted suit with peaked lapels will slim – a double-breasted suit will make you look wider.

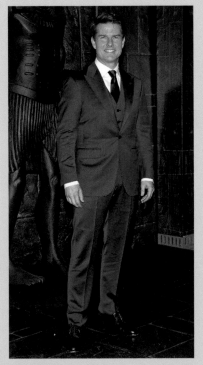

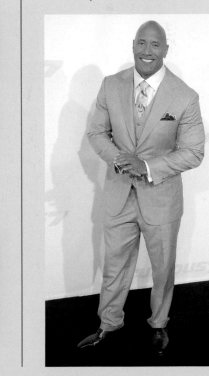

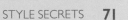

If the suit fits…

Unless you are a very standard size, most suits you buy 'off the rack' will need tweaking by a tailor. A lot of stores will have an alteration service – unless it is free, you might be better off finding someone yourself. Every man needs an alterations tailor. It's a cheap way to look great. Here is a checklist to see whether it's a good fit.

◆ Stand up straight. It's hard to see if something works on you if you are slouching. A good suit will make you want to suck in your gut and stand to attention.

◆ Your number one concern is the jacket. If it doesn't fit well across the chest when buttoned, give it up and walk away. In theory, anything can be altered – in practice, messing with the torso of a suit comes under the category of major surgery.

◆ When you buttoned it, did you breathe in? Are you still breathing in now? Too tight. Try the hug test. Make as if to hug an invisible friend. Does the suit feel like it is about to split at the seams? Walk away.

◆ You want a fit close to your frame but not so snug you can't move. If you can just about slip a flat hand between you and the suit when buttoned, it's a good fit.

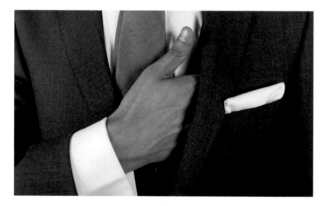

◆ The jacket collar should just touch the neck of the shirt, without a significant gap and with no bunching of material.

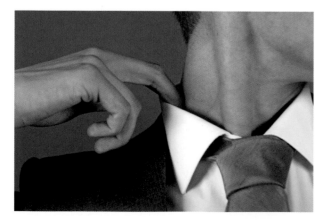

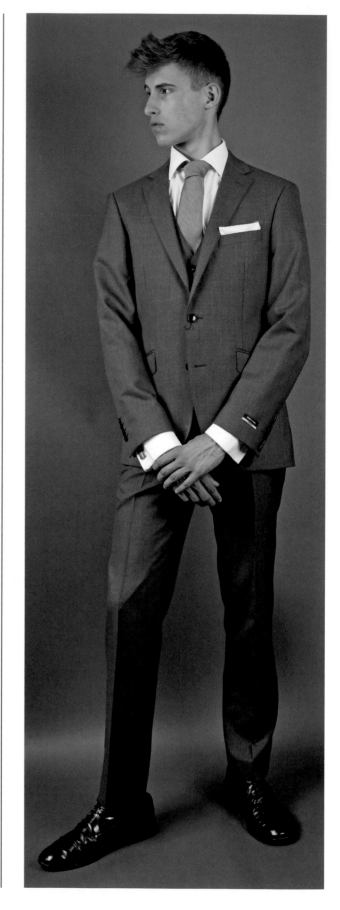

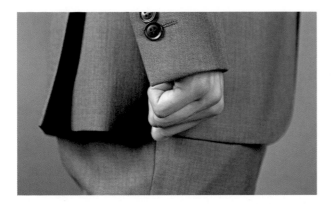

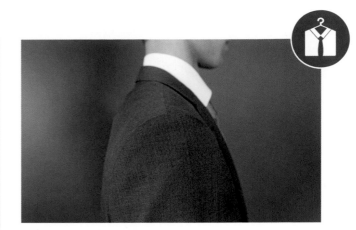

- ◆ Jacket length is vital. Let your arms hang by your sides. Without drawing up your shoulders, bunch your fists. The bottom of the jacket should be about where your knuckles are.
- ◆ Check the view from the back, particularly the seat of the trousers. Too tight will be obvious, and although some men can carry this look, there is a real risk of rippage. Wrinkles and loose material means too big. The ideal is when the fabric touches your underwear but doesn't strain. BTW if the world can clearly see your junk from the front, you need to go up a size.

- ◆ Shoulders should more or less follow the natural line of your own shoulders. If there is a hint of a pinch here, or an overhang of shoulder pad over actual shoulder – walk away. Unless you live in Miami and it is 1985.
- ◆ Two buttons are currently in charge on the high street, but a three-button option always looks sharp. Either way you will not be buttoning the bottom button. A one-button can be carried off by the fashion-forward chap.
- ◆ Jacket sleeves should end where your thumb begins, or just a smidge above the protruding bone of your wrist. This is easily fixed by a tailor. If lengthening is going to be necessary, make sure there is enough material to let out. We should expect to see a bit of shirt cuff – opinions vary on the ideal, but 1cm/1/2in should do.
- ◆ Cuffs can look good on trouser bottoms, especially on a wider leg, but aren't essential. For a traditional length, let the trouser just touch the top of the shoe and crease once.

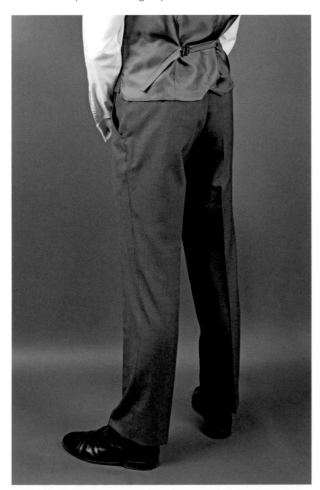

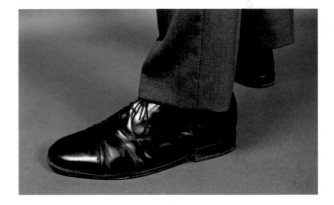

'Clothes don't make a man, but clothes have got many a man a good job'
Herbert Vreeland

Dressing for work

If you work in a trade/a uniform, most of your workday style decisions will be made for you. For everyone else, the workplace can be a sartorial minefield. Even in this more relaxed era, in which many men don't have to wear a suit if they aren't going into meetings, the challenge of choosing an outfit that works is real. There is a lot of freedom, which too many men take as an invitation to put in no effort at all.

To make the most of his career and his image at work, a man has to contrive to fit in while standing out, to excel without being pushy. Happily, it isn't that hard to ace this test.

◆ Do a quick visual survey to check the norms. Are most of your colleagues clean shaven, every day? There's a hint for your morning regimen. Is the guy in accounting the only person in a tie? Maybe you don't need one.

◆ Aim up, not down. There's an old cliché that you should dress for the job you want, not the job you have – corny, but not a bad rule. Put some effort in – go a notch smarter and sharper than the norm/the expectation.

◆ Keep it clean and tidy. There is no excuse, ever, for being at work in clothes that are dirty. Unless you work in the mud-wrestling industry, make this a rule to stick to and always check your clothes thoroughly before stepping out. Ditto creased shirts, lost buttons, frayed hems, trousers worn so often the bum is shiny.

◆ If you hate ironing, buy wrinkle-free or easy-iron clothing. Or pay someone else to do it.

◆ Keep your hygiene levels impeccable. You do not want to be that guy.

◆ If you have a desk or locker, secreting away a spare shirt – along with deodorant and a toothbrush – may one day save your life, or at least your reputation.

◆ Be you. Reflecting the standards you see around you doesn't have to mean dressing exactly like everyone else. Guys in the armed forces should ignore this advice, obvs.

'They say "Dress for the job you want, not the job you have." Now I'm standing in a disciplinary meeting dressed as Batman'

Anon

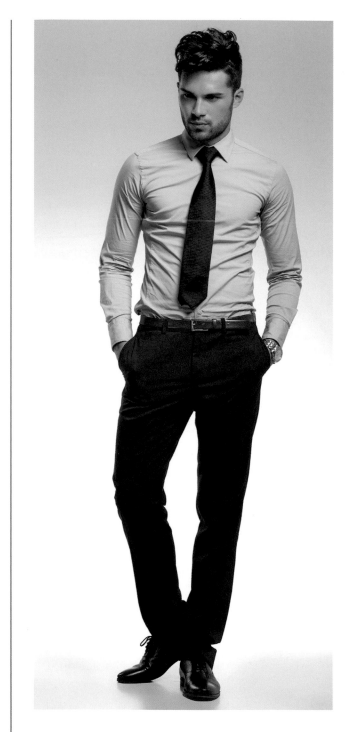

◆ Accessorise. We live in a relaxed, tieless age, which can potentially make the man who does wear a tie the king of the room (though watch for overkill – see previous column re the guy in accounts…). Don't forget good socks, and the power of the pocket square, which works even when you don't have a tie.

◆ Treat yourself to a nice bag, or briefcase – it's a part of your outfit.

◆ Always put your clothes out ready the night before. This will give you time to sort out any issues.

HOW TO
WEAR A POCKET SQUARE

A pocket handkerchief is not for use. Not for sneezing into, not for removing lipstick, not even for someone's tears – unless this is a very extreme situation and you are fully in love. Keep a clean white hanky somewhere else for these moments – tucked up your sleeve is handy. 'One for blowing, one for showing' is the rule.

Your pocket square can be plain white, to match a white shirt, or something else entirely. If the rest of your outfit is fairly sober, you can really go for this. Try to make it echo something else about your outfit – colour, texture – but avoid aiming for a very precise match.

There are many ways of wearing a pocket square, but they boil down to the precise approach – rectangle, sharp points – or louche – a 'puff' or loose points. Which you choose is up to you, and there's room for improvisation, but the latter is arguably a little more confident/ stylish, while the former suits a white handkerchief and an uptight, crisp Mad Men look.

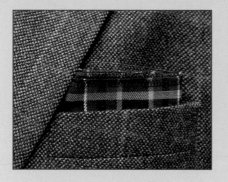

Rectangle
A precise rectangle is easy to achieve – fold the hanky to the width of the pocket, and iron it into shape.

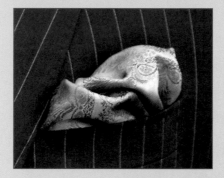

The puff
Hold the middle of the square, put the finger and thumb of your other hand together and push the hanky through the hole. Insert into pocket, puff side up, tuck away any spare bits as you do.

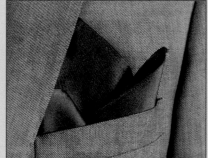

Three-point
The classic shape, this can work in precise or louche mode.

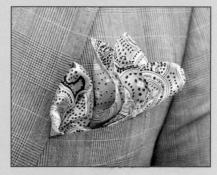

The whatever
Hold the middle of the square, and tuck it in to the pocket puff side down, with lots of corners showing. Adjust to suit, or leave it wild.

How to fold a Three-point

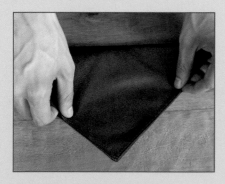

1 Fold the hanky on a flat surface once across the middle into a triangle, with the point at the top.

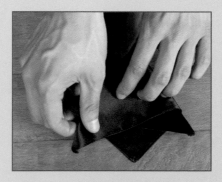

2 Then fold both the left and right corners up to form points to the left and right of the main peak.

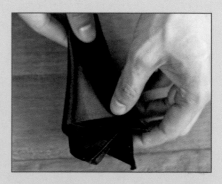

3 Turn the square over and fold left and right sides again to make an ice-cream cone. Tuck it into place.

STYLE RULES

Men's clothing comes with lots of golden rules – what you should never do, in any circumstances, and what you must always do, every time. This freaks a lot of men out, and with good reason. Too many people who are into clothes rely too heavily on those stipulations – forgetting that this takes most of the fun out of it. Men may be tempted to take the safer option, and stick with what they feel comfortable with, take no risks.

The point, however, is not to stick to the rules slavishly, but to learn from them. Because most of them aren't entirely arbitrary. Often, they exist for a good reason – the product of generations of male wisdom, passed down from chaps who really knew clothes – and are intended to ensure you look your best. So before you break the rules, the least you can do is to take a moment to reflect on them.

1 Watch out for crimes against colour

There are a number of colour combinations that, on paper at least, are supposed to be off-limits – usually for the very good reason that they have the potential to look terrible together. Blue and black, for example, can be difficult to pull off – too alike to offer contrast and too different to match. White and cream is a similarly fraught question. Another rule says 'brown and green should never be seen', which is good advice – I once tried to combine brown chinos with a green polo neck, only to be told that I looked like a tree. Which was fair criticism.

When to break it
Whenever you feel like it. Seriously, it can be good to do the things with colour you are not supposed to do – and sometimes it works precisely because it shouldn't. But if in doubt (and if you are one of the 8% of men who are colour blind) get a second opinion.

2 The hem of your trouser should touch the top of your shoe

… and the fabric should 'break', in one small indentation. This rule is flexible depending on the width of the trouser, the material, etc and the trend recently has been towards a higher hem – but the fundamental position is still the best place to start, particularly with a suit, or smarter trousers. This is designed to ensure you have the correct amount of sock/ankle showing when standing and when sitting. Too much trouser and it will puddle, making you look like you are borrowing a grown-up's outfit for the day. Too little trouser and you risk exposing your hairy calves to the world, though of course you may choose to adopt the rolled-up or cropped look.

When to break it
The rule is flexible, depending on the trouser and what's underneath it. If you have the nerve, by all means go for the nerdish look and expose a bit of sock, for instance by rolling up a chino, or ditch the socks entirely and pair turned-up jeans with old-school trainers/sneakers… For smarter trousers or a suit, a good halfway solution is a trouser that only just touches the top of the shoe.

'With a suit, always wear big British shoes, the ones with large welts. There's nothing worse than dainty little Italian jobs at the end of the leg line'
David Bowie

3 Avoid the male tail

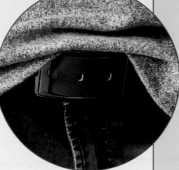

The problem: trousers that fall off your hips, so that when you bend over you gift the world a sight of your underwear, or worse. I'm not saying that no one wants to see your arse. I'm sure there is a market for it. But time and place, man, time and place. The time is not now, and the place is not someone's kitchen while you attempt to fix the sink.

When to break it
Never. It isn't flattering or practical, and odds are you will be judged accordingly. If you want to look like a grown man, buy a belt.

4 Never wear a black belt with brown shoes

This one is easy: aim to wear the same colour belt as your shoes. You don't have to go crazy 'matchy-matchy' with it, and a complementing colour works – but never, ever black belt, brown shoes, or vice versa.

When to break it
Never. See above. You can still do an interesting belt – canvas, navy, whatever – but you can't break the brown/black rule.

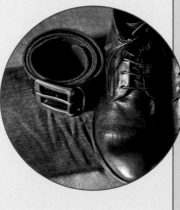

5 Don't/Do wear brown shoes in the office

There is considerable confusion about when a brown shoe can be worn safely. Some have misunderstood the (very dated) rules about 'no brown in town' to mean that you ought never to wear a brown shoe with a suit, or to work. In fact this depends entirely on the suit, and the workplace. If yours is a very formal, old-fashioned work environment (eg banking) the black shoe is generally going to be the safer option. But with many suits – dark blue, mid-grey, brown, tan – a dark-brown shoe works very well, and adds interest to your outfit.

When to break it
You can absolutely wear brown shoes in a whole host of different contexts (including the office) but take care that it works with the setting and the rest of your attire. The more formal the outfit or the occasion, the more likely that black will be the safer bet. Darker browns are more flexible and easier to match and light/tan shoes are really for the summer only.

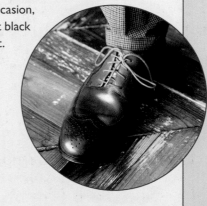

'Your socks have got to be long enough so you don't have a big expanse of leg between your trouser top and your socks … you wouldn't even need to explain that to an Italian'
Alan Johnson

WEDDING WEAR 101

Dressing for a major life event can make a man feel like he is staring down the barrel of a loaded gun. The choice of outfit represents all of the other pressures bearing down on the groom: in-laws; expenses; a partner who is noticeably more insane as the big day approaches. Take heart. Done right, this process can be fun and can leave you with a happy spouse, a great outfit you'll wear again and wedding pictures to be proud of.

Do not ask the bride/groom to choose

If there is a wedding theme, you certainly want to reflect it, and there is nothing wrong with hearing your partner's views on what the ideal groom should look like – if you are gay, your soon-to-be-husband will hopefully have given it a lot of thought too. However, inviting your fiancée to select your wedding outfit is like having your mum accompany you to buy underwear. Stand up, and choose your own trousers. There is one very important caveat to this rule:

Do ask someone else for their opinion

Someone from your partner's side, intimately connected to the wedding planning, can at least give you an idea of what not to wear, colours to avoid, that sort of thing. If there is

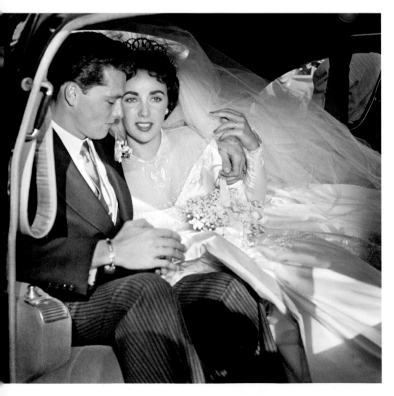

no one else, and the bride/groom is on the total control side of things, then ignore rule 1 – but remember, you are looking for guidance, not a shopping list.

Don't leave it late

Delaying this is the mistake most likely to leave you looking foolish on the big day. Give yourself months, not weeks – and certainly not days – to get this right.

Don't forget a wingman

This is too big a deal to go through on your own. Ask the best-dressed man you know to accompany you shopping, to give you an honest answer on what makes you look good and what doesn't. He doesn't have to be the Best Man – just the best man for this job. He may also discreetly leak a picture of your outfit to your partner, just to make sure they're happy.

Do buy, don't rent

Your partner may have pictured a wedding photo in which all the men are wearing identical maroon tuxedos. If not, then take our advice and let the best man, father of the bride, etc sort out their own outfits. Not your problem. Rented suits will never fit perfectly – whereas if you buy, you'll get a classy outfit, altered to fit, that is yours for life. If you do want the men to have something in common, you can do it subtly – with matching ties, boutonnières or pocket squares.

Context, context, context

What you wear depends on a huge range of factors – where you are getting married, when (season, time of day), and to whom. We've suggested below the perfect Swiss-army-knife outfit, which will do you for most eventualities, including church, town hall and garden weddings. However, if you are planning on getting married on a boat, a beach, or the bridge of the *USS Enterprise*, clearly there is room for a different approach.

Don't assume you need a tailor

If you are dropping serious cash, and can afford to, there is a strong argument for getting something tailor made, bespoke, just for you. However, bear in mind this is not a good time for untested ideas. There is a lot of pressure, a lot can be lost in translation, and a suit that only gets worn once is a waste of money. If you do go bespoke, make sure you can trust your tailor to deliver what you want.

Do follow the rules

There are many rules about formal menswear for weddings. Some of them make sense, some don't, and some are only needed by minor royalty. There are however two good rules of thumb for the real world:

◆ Tuxedos are for the evening. If you are getting married in daylight hours, the Cary Grant look is out.
◆ Formal day wear (the super-posh world of top hats and tailcoats) is very, very difficult to get right. For 99% of men the minefield of acceptable lapels, collars, gloves, etc is going to be way too much work. Of course, you can always rent – see opposite for reasons why not.

Do buy a dark lounge suit

It doesn't sound particularly exciting, but the quality dark lounge suit is the single most important must-have item in any man's sartorial life – suitable for weddings, funerals, court appearances, job interviews, divorce proceedings, second weddings (joke) and more.

➤ This suit is the one. Make sure it feels right.

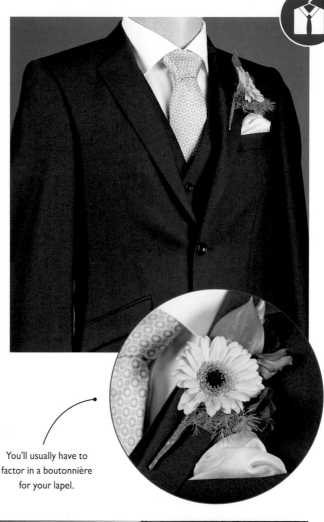

You'll usually have to factor in a boutonnière for your lapel.

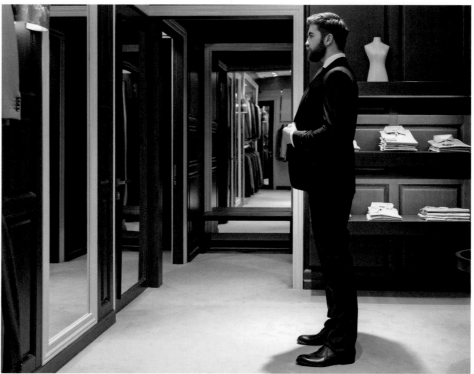

'A man should look as if he's bought his clothes with intelligence, put them on with care and then forgotten all about them'
Hardy Amies

Don't, just don't…

Wear garish, brightly coloured waistcoats, pre-tied cravats, clip-on bow ties, black work socks, old underwear (at least one person will be seeing these. Treat yourself). Brown shoes are generally a no, unless you and she are going rustic chic – they may work with tweed for an outdoor wedding, for instance.

Do wear any colour (as long as it is blue or grey)

You want this suit to go with everything, to make you look smart but not overshadow your partner, so keep it simple. It is not possible to go wrong with dark blue or grey – flattering, classic looks that work well in all kinds of settings and a range of skin tones. If that feels a little safe, try very light grey, or a steely mid-blue. A stripe or other pattern is a possibility, but make sure it is discreet – very small micro-patterns work best.

Do buy the best (you can afford)

This is an opportunity to splash out, within your means. Look online or in men's style mags to see which names float your boat. Ideally, go for something in high-quality wool, suitable for the climate. You will be wearing this all day, so don't choose a lightweight summer fabric for a church hall in January, or heavy wool for August in St Tropez. You can get more for your money buying from an outlet centre or in the sales – winter suits will be cheaper in the spring, and vice versa. See p68 for more on buying a suit.

▼ You can afford to splash more flash than usual.

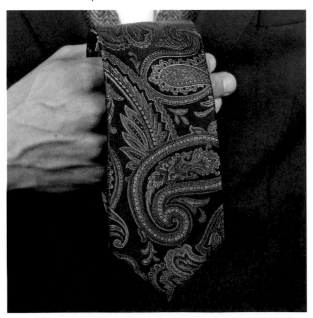

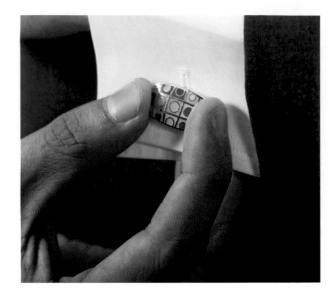

▲ French cuffs are a must; be sure to rock a good cufflink.

Do make sure it fits

The cut is up to you and your body type, but the fit should be immaculate. For most men, single-breasted is a safe bet that gives you options, but the formality of the wedding context means you can think about trying double-breasted. Remember you are aiming to flatter yourself with a style that gives you a good silhouette, a narrow waist and a strong shoulder.

When trying on, wear the shoes you will wear to the wedding and a shirt and tie – it'll give you a sense of what the finished look might be. Make sure you leave time for alterations. Sleeves and trouser legs are easily fixed – anything more major, leave it on the rack. You want a fit that is close enough to flatter, but not so tight you'll be sucking in your stomach all day. See p72 for guidance on fit.

Do primp

Get your hair done (tell the hairdresser it's your wedding cut – it'll keep them focused), shave with a new razor, get your teeth whitened, go to the gym, eat well, stop drinking, get some sun/air/sleep – do whatever it takes in the days and weeks before the big day to get you looking and feeling good.

And finally… don't forget to be yourself

The feeling you are aiming for here is you, at your best. If you feel instead like a plum in a rented Halloween costume, you are entitled to change the look. However, before freaking out, you would do well to remember that you're just the straight man in this act – the audience are here for her, and your role is to look your best, say yes at the right moments, and look after her. Welcome to married life.

ACCESSORIES

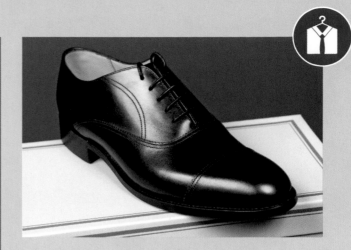

This is where the fun starts – where you lift your outfit from the everyday to the splendid, and start to look like a man on his way to the most important fixture of his life. Indulge yourself, shop around, use your imagination and get some advice – this is a good excuse to get out of the way during the stressful wedding prep period.

◆ Shirt: Buy the nicest white shirt you can afford, with French cuffs for cufflinks and a collar wide enough to take the tie you will go for. Try it with the jacket to make sure they work together. Make sure the collar in particular is a perfect fit – not so tight you feel strangled, and not so loose there is a visible gap.

◆ Boutonnière: The flower you will wear in your lapel, to be coordinated with any wedding flower theme. Usually collected from the church/venue. If you don't have a working buttonhole it can be pinned in place.

◆ Waistcoat: Buying a suit that comes with a waistcoat (a three-piece) is a simple way to make yourself super-smart. A non-matching waistcoat is a risky proposition that may – or may not – come off. Better to play it safe.

◆ Tie: As lavish and silky as possible. Silver/grey is a good option – go for something jazzier than you might wear at work, but not totally OTT. A cravat is a possibility, but can look slightly ridiculous with a lounge suit – a good tie is a safer option.

◆ Pocket square: A splash of colour and texture that should complement the tie – but doesn't have to match it precisely. If you can get something that mirrors your bride's dress, well done you.

◆ Socks: These could be something more than plain black, but not a crazy novelty colour or design. Coordinate with tie and/or wedding colour theme.

◆ Shoes: **Do not wear old work shoes.** Spring for a new pair, ideally black, highly polished. Lace-up, cap-toed, ideally, but a classic pair of Chelsea boots can also work. Not super-chunky heavy brogues, unless you are marrying in a field. As noted, black is more classic than brown, which is more suitable for an outdoors or rural wedding. Break them in a bit before the day – you are likely to spend most of it standing and some of it dancing.

◆ Belt: If your trousers need a belt, buy one that is good quality, subtle and in a colour that matches or complements your shoes. For bonus points, any metal should match your cufflinks. Suspenders may also be an option.

◆ Jewellery: A wedding ring, obviously, but there may also be room for a little sparkle – cufflinks, alongside a vintage stick-pin or tie bar to hold your neckwear in place.

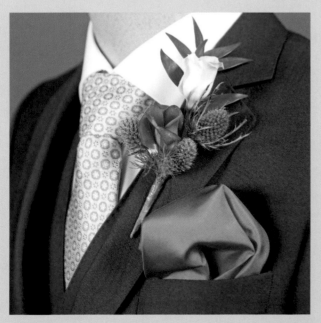

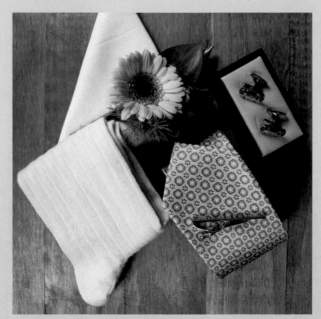

WEARING A TUX

You are unlikely to own more than one tux, if that, or to wear it more than once in a blue moon, so you can expect it to last. A tuxedo you own, which really fits you, is a gift that will keep on giving you the edge over the fellow in the rental. It is possible to go leftfield with this choice, to push the boundaries of colour and cut – but when the classic number does the job so well, it makes more sense to invest accordingly.

Equipment

Tuxedo, white shirt with French cuffs and some detailing, bow tie, cummerbund (optional), black Oxford shoes, braces/suspenders (optional), black socks.

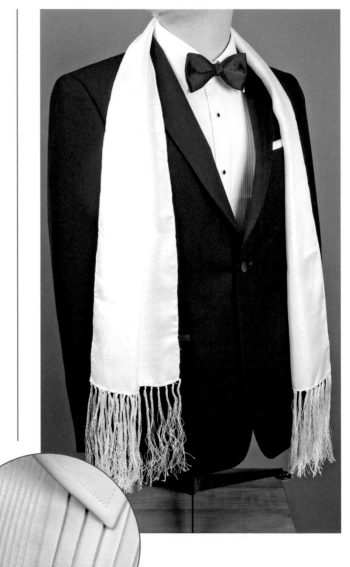

White shirt with French cuffs and not a wing collar.

◆ A tux usually has a black or midnight-blue jacket with peak or shawl lapels and, traditionally, no vent at the back or side vents, to keep the line clean. The quality of the fabric matters – barathea, mohair and velvet are the crème de la crème.

◆ A white (actually ivory/cream) jacket is possible – traditionally reserved for summer or hot climates. For how to rock this look, see James Bond.

◆ White shirt with French cuffs and some sort of detailing – most likely, pleats. Ruffles are for the brave. Not a wing collar!

◆ Bow tie. Learn how to tie your own – so much more impressive than a pre-tied one or, even worse, a clip-on.

◆ Cummerbund – not essential, but this sash for your waist covers up the trouser/shirt boundary with style. Usually black, in a fabric that matches the lapels. Pleats go upwards. Consider instead a waistcoat to conceal the waist and bring elegance – this is more than a simple suit. Or go double-breasted.

◆ Well-shined black Oxford shoes. Patent are very acceptable but not vital. The truly bold, who aren't going to be taking the night bus home, can go for evening shoes – sleek little slippers with a pretty bow on top.

◆ Braces, or suspenders – if you need to hold up the trousers, this is how. Ideally fastened with buttons, rather than being of the clip-on variety. Never, ever wear a belt with a tuxedo.

◆ Trousers match the jacket, and have a braid stripe on the side. No cuffs, ever, and no pleats, mostly.

◆ Black socks are best.

HOW TO
TIE A BOW TIE

Once the province of antique dealers and nerds in high-school movies, the bow tie has recently made an unexpected comeback. There is no possible justification for wearing a pre-tied or clip-on bow tie, so learn to do it the hard way. Tying one is a fiddly affair, so stick with it – practice makes perfect.

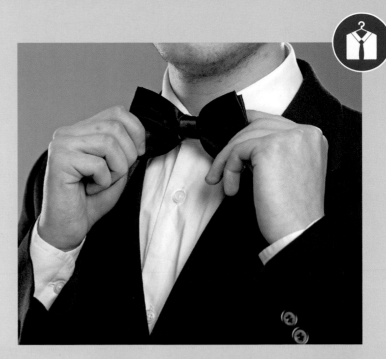

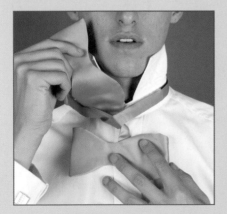

1 A bow tie is a challenge, but you can handle it. Be sure you didn't buy pre-tied.

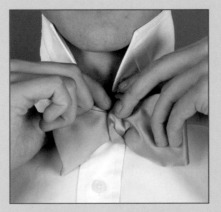

2 Drape around your neck, one end slightly longer than the other.

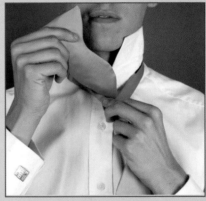

3 Tuck the long end of the tie under the other and loop it over.

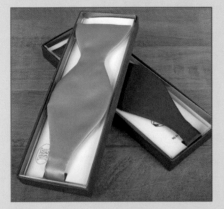

4 Fiddly bit. Make a bow shape with the shorter end by folding it. Bring the long end straight down over it.

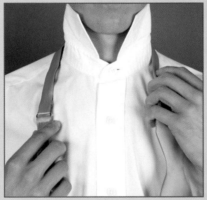

5 Fold the long bit into a bow shape, pinch it tight, and tuck the pinched bit in behind the first bow, through the loop you made when you brought it over. Curse, loudly.

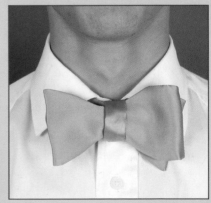

6 You thought you'd never get here, but you made it. Pull gently on the folded bits to tighten and straighten.

MEN'S STYLING SECRETS

The world of men's style contains many, many rules and processes, some of which can seem both exhausting and pointless. It's entirely possible to look good with relatively little effort, and some perfectly stylish guys may choose to ignore the rules entirely and do their own thing. However, if you think you might want to draw on the accumulated knowledge of generations of stylish gents, it's a good idea to learn and perfect a few old-school skills.

What to wear when

Different occasions call for different clothes – you don't want to go clubbing or to a festival in a muddy field wearing a three-piece suit, and turning up to a funeral in a velour tracksuit will get you funny looks. In a world of men's style which is increasingly casual, there is great flexibility, but the ideas below should help you gauge what sort of thing is generally acceptable in particular situations.

Trying to interpret the dress code for an event can be another sartorial minefield, particularly where the host has tried to sum it up with a shorthand phrase that may not mean much to you. If you are in any doubt about what to wear, ask the host – better to bother them with questions than turn up to the BBQ in white tie and tails.

A job interview

You are looking to make an instant impression, so your ideal interview outfit is smart, focused, detail oriented, clean and sharp – all the qualities you are trying to project. Look at the dress code in the workplace and aim slightly higher. If suits and open shirts are the norm, wear a tie. Reign in the urge to be flashy – the odds are that a dark suit in a solid, unpatterned blue or grey will be your best bet, with a (new, or newish) white shirt and a good tie. If you get a second interview, it's OK to repeat the suit, but change the tie. Black, well-polished lace-up shoes are a solid option with an interview suit, but brown can also work, especially if you aren't trying to get a job in banking. If you don't own a suit, go for the smartest outfit you have, immaculately clean and pressed.

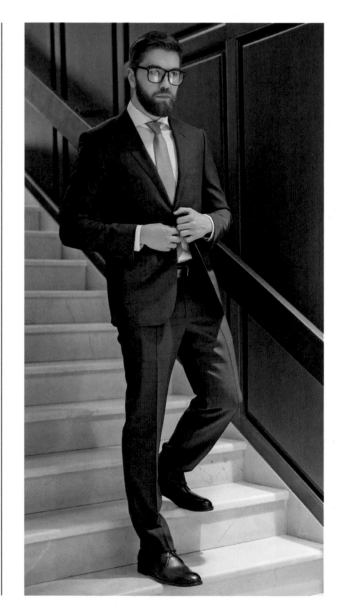

DECODE THE DRESS CODE

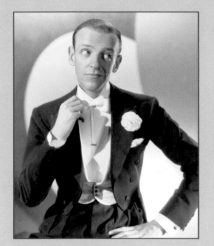

White tie

Top of the line in terms of formality, white tie means black tailcoat, black trousers, white waistcoat, wing-collar shirt. Frankly if you live a life that involves regular white-tie events, you probably have all this – and if you don't, you'll be renting from someone who will kit you out.

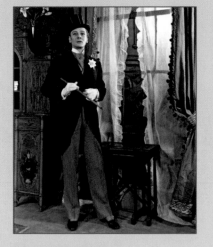

Morning dress

Morning coat in grey or black with tails, black/striped trousers, light grey waistcoat, turn-down collared shirt, cravat, top hat. The daytime version of formal white tie, with similarly strict rules and impeccable standards likely to be enforced.

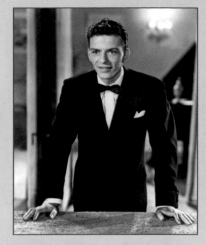

Black tie/semi-formal/ Evening dress

Tuxedo, basically. 'Black tie optional' means wear a tux or feel underdressed. (See p82 for more on the rules of the tuxedo.) In general it's best to avoid wearing a regular black tie with a tuxedo, AKA a Hollywood Tux.

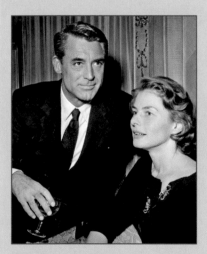

Cocktail attire

More common in the US, this is a vague term, open to interpretation. In general the mood is semi-formal, halfway between a day at the office and a posh night out. The precise look depends on the setting, but for evenings, a super sharp and understated dark suit would work, tieless or otherwise.

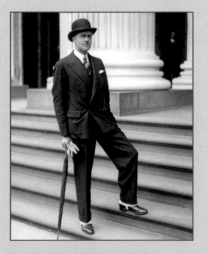

Business attire

A smart suit, with tie. Turn it up a notch from regular work wear, if you can – good excuse to buy a new tie. If the event looks like it might be on the sober end of the spectrum, keep it formal and keep flash (jewellery, sporty shoes, pungent aftershave) to a minimum.

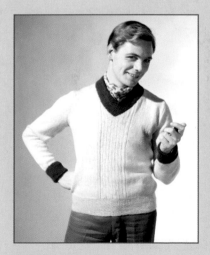

Smart casual

Oxymoronic shorthand for 'look presentable'. There is no universally agreed meaning for 'smart casual', but if you pitch it smart but not over-fussy, you won't go far wrong. You don't need a tie, or a suit, but a blazer is good. Denim may be too casual, but a pair of well fitting chinos will do the job.

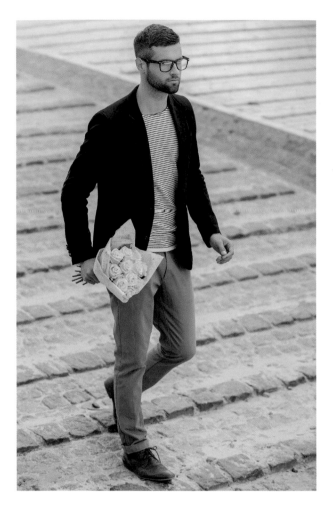

Meet the parents

If you are crossing this line it is likely there is some future to the relationship – you don't want to blow this with a bad first impression. You are aiming to be yourself, but with a heavy emphasis on projecting the fact that you are approachable, reliable and stable. The kind of man you would trust to look after your offspring. Go sensible, go smart but relaxed, shave, brush your hair, go easy on the cologne.

A funeral

Don't worry about looking good – that isn't the point. Wear a dark suit, black if you have it, grey or dark blue if not. A black tie, either way. Eschew the usual details, like pocket square, jewellery, etc – any flash in this context is inappropriate. Make sure you are clean and pressed and shoes are polished – it is disrespectful to the family and the deceased not to put in a bit of effort.

Someone else's wedding

You are not the star of this show. But you are going to be in all the pictures, so put your back into it. Particularly if you happen to be single… A good suit works, and if it is in the summer, go for lightweight linens and experiment with lighter colours. Accessorise with a snappy hat – a trilby or similar with a stingy brim (Google it) is good – remember to take it off during the ceremony.

A first date

On a first date, it doesn't hurt to let it show that you put in some work. Dress with care, and appropriately for the venue, but don't overdo it – unless the restaurant is four star, a suit and tie is going to be overkill. A contrasting suit jacket (AKA 'sport coat') is appropriate in many settings, particularly with dark, slim denim, while soft, quality knitwear is supremely tactile. This is a good moment to wheel out a signature piece/favourite garment – and if you don't have something that meets that description, a good excuse to buy one. It goes without saying that your hygiene and grooming should be beyond reproach. Ditto shoes – don't let the outfit down with lazy, scuffed footwear, because it will probably be checked. And wear your very best pants, just in case.

'If you can't be better than your competition, just dress better'
Anna Wintour

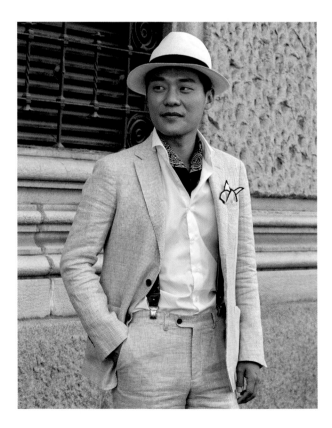

HOW TO
TIE A FOUR-IN-HAND KNOT

There are at least 400 ways to tie a tie, but you don't need to know 397 of them. The main difference in styles is the size and evenness of the knot – your choice depends on the tie, the shirt collar and the suit.

The classic everyday knot is the four-in-hand. This is reasonably slender, easy to tie, and works with most shirt collars, apart from a wide, spread collar – against which it will look insignificant.

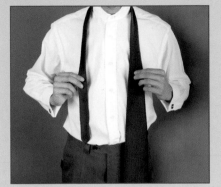

1 Place tie around neck, making sure the wider end dangles a few inches below the narrow end.

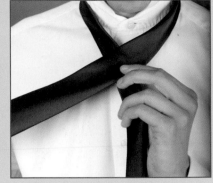

2 Bring the fat end over the thin end once.

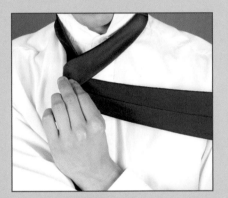

3 And then loop the fat end under the thin.

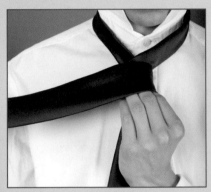

4 Bring it round again, and then under, creating a little gap – leave a finger or two in there.

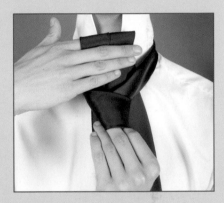

5 Bring the fat end under the knot, next to your shirt/neck.

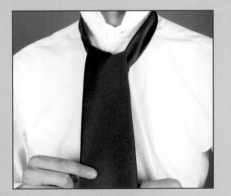

6 Pull it through so it flops back over, sitting on top of the knot.

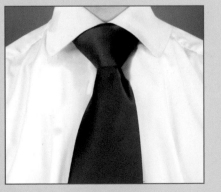

7 Tuck the fat end through the gap you made earlier. Pull on the fat end to tighten and adjust the knot to suit your shirt. Leave a dimple in the knot.

Length

The fat end of the tie should always be marginally longer than the narrow end. Length depends on the tie and the suit, but a very general rule of thumb is for it to end around where your belt's button holes are, while you are standing normally. If the end of the tie dangles somewhere around your trouser fly, it is too long – try a different knot. Don't tuck it in.

HOW TO TIE A WINDSOR KNOT

Shirts with a wider, spread collar need a thicker, triangular knot to look their best. The Windsor was made to emulate the style of the nattiest dresser of his era, the Duke of Windsor (who had his ties made extra thick for a fatter knot). It doesn't matter which end goes to the left/right, as long as you are consistent.

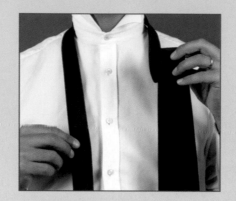

1 Start with your collar up and buttoned, tie draped around your neck. Leave the fat end of the tie longer than the narrow end.

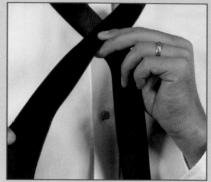

2 Bring the fat end over the narrow, making an X – the start of the knot.

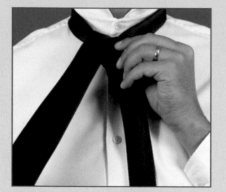

3 Loop the fat end in under the narrow and then out again, letting it fall to the same side it went in.

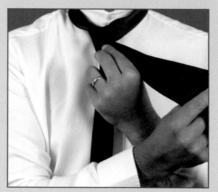

4 Wrap it around once behind the narrow end and back again to make a knot. The underside of the fat end should be visible.

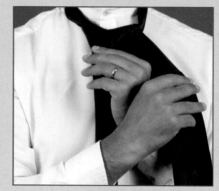

5 Push the fat end through the neck loop and down to the other side, so the underside is showing again. The unfinished knot is now starting to look even/triangular.

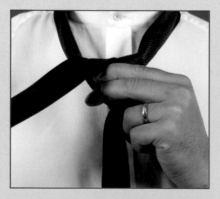

6 Wrap the fat end over the knot, so the front shows again, then pull it up through the neck loop.

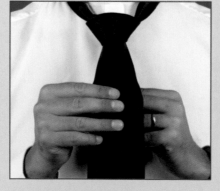

7 Drape the fat end over, then tuck it in to make the knot.

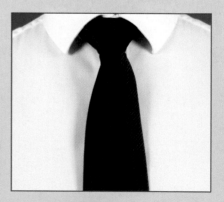

8 Tug gently on the wide end to tighten the knot, use both hands to shift it up to your collar.

HOW TO
TIE A HALF-WINDSOR KNOT

A good medium-sized knot, suitable for all sorts of contexts. Neat and tidy, it works with medium and light fabrics and may not suit a very thick tie. Tie to the left or the right, but keep it consistent/even.

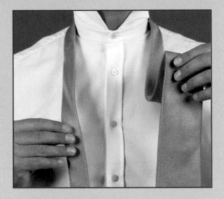

1 Start with your shirt collar up and buttoned. Leave the fat end of the tie several inches longer than the narrow end.

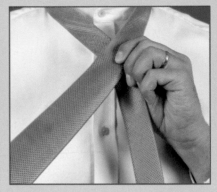

2 Place the fat end over the narrow end, making an X which will be the start of your knot.

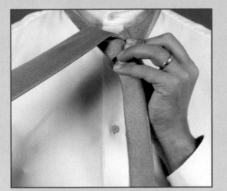

3 Loop it around the back, into the space between collar and tie and out again, hanging to the same side it was before.

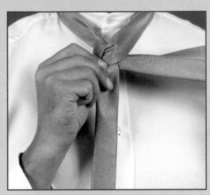

4 Wrap the fat end round the back behind the knot, underside showing.

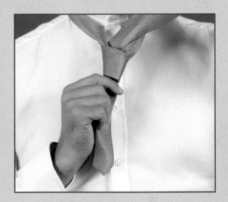

5 Then back over the knot and into the neck loop, so the underside is showing again. Don't pull it tight yet.

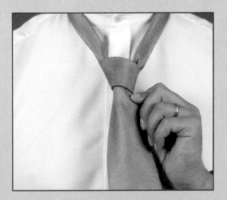

6 Pull the fat end over the front of the knot and back behind, then push/pull the fat end through the loop you just made.

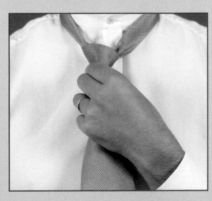

7 Tighten by pulling gently and sliding the knot up towards the collar.

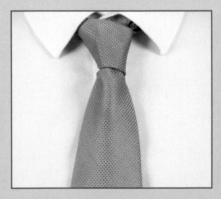

8 The finished job should look neat and triangular – for bonus points, aim for a dimple just under the knot.

CARING FOR YOUR CLOTHES

Nothing lets down an outfit like shoddy care. Italian men are generally acknowledged as the best-dressed chaps in the world – not just because of their effortless style, but also in their approach to caring for their clothes. Garments are respected, cleaned, pressed, brushed, so that even the most humble outfit puts on a good show. It costs nothing to look after your clothes properly – just a little time and effort.

Suit care

Suits – and blazers/sports coats, and smart trousers – need looking after, or they won't go the distance. Buy a clothes brush and sturdy wooden hangers. Cedar-wood blocks are a good investment, putting off moths without the stink of chemicals, while garment bags protect suits and jackets from dust.

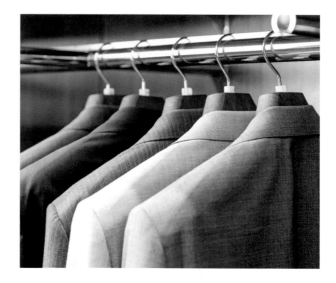

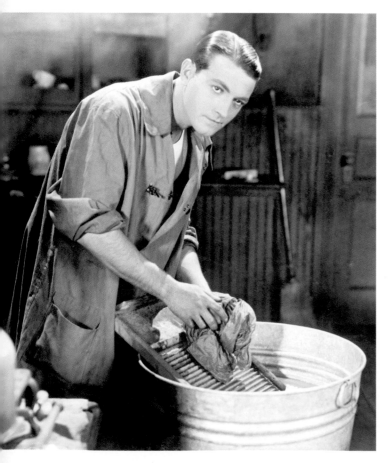

If you wear a suit regularly, get in the habit of taking it off when you get home, rather than lounging around in it. Hang it from a wooden hanger, taking care that the fold respects the creases in the trousers, and that pockets are empty. Give it a brush, especially the shoulder areas. Let it air a bit before hanging away in a garment bag. Leave it a couple of days before wearing it again, if you can, to give it time to recover.

Dry-cleaning should be an annual event, not something that happens every week or month. The harsh chemicals involved are not good for the suit, or the planet. Instead, give it a regular brush, with an occasional steam and if it needs it, a very gentle press (a steam cleaner is a cheap and useful tool). When on the road, and without a trouser press or similar, resort to the travelling salesman's trick for removing wrinkles: turn the hotel shower on hot, hang the suit up, close the door. A good 10-minute steam should restore a bit of shape.

HOW TO
IRON A SHIRT

Some people find ironing shirts soothing, most don't. You can make it significantly less tiresome in one of three ways:

1 Learn to do it properly.
2 Buy shirts that need little ironing. Shop carefully, because some easy-care shirts look like easy-care shirts. Convenience is the enemy of style.
3 Get someone else to do it.

If taking option 1, equip yourself with a decent steam iron and an ironing board set to the right height. If you don't have room for a full-size board, you can get something that sits on the table. Don't even try attempting this with a floor and a towel.

Fill the iron with water and let it heat to the temperature advised on the shirt label. Use smooth strokes, gentle pressure – and take care in laying the shirt on the board. Hit the 'steam' button liberally – think of it as a turbo boost. The spray from the front is for the stubborn and sensitive areas. This is the right order in which to iron your shirt. Other orders are available, but they are wrong. Make the ironing process easier by prepping – when the shirt comes out of the dryer, hang it up straight away. If line drying, use a hanger.

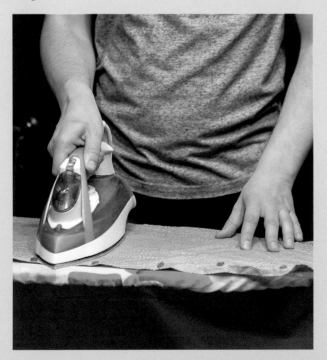

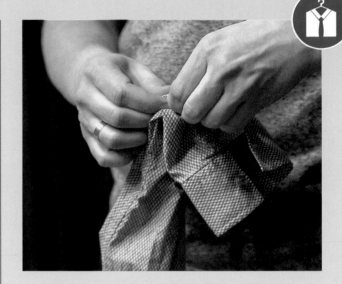

Equipment
Steam iron, ironing board, shirt.

1 Lay the collar out carefully, iron the back first, then the front. Lay the yoke/shoulders of the shirt carefully on the board, inserting the narrow end into a shoulder. Iron each shoulder section.

3 Sleeves next. Lay each arm out one at a time, carefully, buttons/cuff-link holes facing up, with the fold along the hem. Any folds you leave will be ironed in, so take the time to get this right. Sleeves don't have to have a hard crease, unless you want one. If so, pass the iron across for a straight line – if not, iron close to the top edge before flipping over. Always iron both sides of a sleeve. Then the cuffs, laying them out open (you don't want a crease in your cuffs).

4 Next is the body – buttonhole side first, then all the way around via the back. Iron around buttons, hitting the steam/spray buttons as necessary. Never iron on top of the buttons – this will damage them.

5 Done. Hang up the shirt immediately, buttoning up the top button.

'I realize how talented our hair and wardrobe people are every time I have to get dressed on my own'
Jon Hamm

HOW TO
SEW ON A BUTTON

Sewing on a button is easy. You'll need a pin (or matchstick/toothpick), needle and thread. The colour of the thread will be determined by that used on the other buttons – generally, something discreet. Work out where the button needs to be by locating the old holes.

1 Thread the needle. Pull a few inches of thread through, an equal amount on both sides. Cut, then tie a knot to keep the stray ends together.
2 Do a couple of stitches to keep the thread secure – push the needle through the fabric in the right place and back again.
3 Hold the button in place, then push the needle through the fabric and through one of the button holes. Pull until the knot is braced against the fabric.
4 Lay a pin/matchstick/toothpick across the middle of the button. This keeps it from being stitched too tightly, which makes doing it up tricky once it has been sewn on. Push the needle back through the fabric, opposite where it came out.
5 Repeat the last two steps until the button feels secure – at least four times for a shirt, eight or more for a jacket. If you are stitching a four-hole button, copy how the other buttons are stitched (crossed or parallel stitches).
6 To finish, push the needle through from the back again, but instead of putting it through the button, pull it to the side.
7 Remove the pin, then start to wrap the thread around the stitches you created, between the button and the fabric, keeping it nice and tight.
8 Push the needle back through the button then back again to the back of the fabric. Flip over the material and finish off the job by making a few stitches between the shirt and button. Cut the thread, and tie it off.
9 Snip off any excess thread.

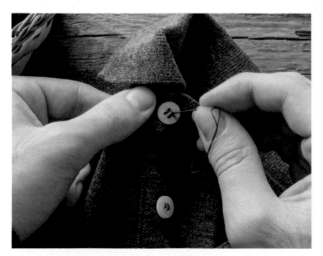

HOW TO
PACK A SUITCASE

Where are you going, and for how long? What's the weather forecast? Are you going to be able to wash and re-wear clothes there? Will you be visiting fancy restaurants, or beach bars? Traipsing around cobbled streets, or hiking steep hills?

In most scenarios it's best to take light clothes that will do duty for any eventuality, and can be layered. Good wool sweaters in merino or cashmere are unbeatable. For colder climates, thermal underclothes and a down jacket will help you travel light. Footwear is a very important call – if you are bringing sturdy boots or other bulky items, save packing space by wearing them for the journey.

Make sure everything is clean and pressed – it is way easier to pack ironed clothes. Lay everything out on the bed. Review everything – does it all more or less match? The most common mistake is over-packing, so be ruthless. In a pinch you can always wash a shirt and wear it again.

◆ The heaviest stuff goes at the bottom. If it's a wheely suitcase, make sure heavy shoes, books, etc are by the wheels.
◆ Stuff socks, underwear, etc into shoes. If you are bringing a tie, roll it tightly and insert it into a (not smelly) shoe. Wrap footwear in plastic bags and lay them at the bottom (the plastic bags will do for dirty laundry when you get there).
◆ Some clothes can be rolled tightly – T-shirts and anything that doesn't wrinkle, such as jeans. Lay these over the shoe layer. Leave a small gap in the middle and place your toiletries bag there.
◆ Fold shirts, suit jackets, etc and lay them over the rolled layer. Trousers should be folded in half and laid across the length of the bag. They are thicker at the waist, so alternate the direction in which you place them.
◆ Folding suit jackets:

1 Holding the top of the jacket in both hands, turn it inside out at one shoulder.
2 Fold the other shoulder into the space created.
3 Draw the sides together so the whole jacket is as wide as the shoulder.
4 Fold it in half over your arm so it is now quartered, in a square shape, the shoulder lining up with the jacket bottom.
5 Place it in a plastic bag – a resealable giant zipped suit one is perfect, otherwise a carrier bag.
6 Lay the jacket carefully in the suitcase. If you place it flat with folded items on top of it (not awkward bits such as shoes) it will be less likely to move about and wrinkle.

HOW TO
CLEAN SHOES

Polishing shoes

Get the right polish for the shoe. A cobbler will be able to recommend a good product – ask their advice. Your choices include wax and cream – liquid polishes dispensed via a little sponge are convenient but don't do anything to protect the leather, and won't get you a nice deep shine. Shoe polishes come in a range of colours – aim for a good match, but if you are unsure, buy neutral.

Equipment

Polish, shoe brush, cloth (eg an old T-shirt), newspaper.

1 Put down newspaper. Polish stains everything. Brush away any dirt on the shoe with a stiff brush or a slightly damp cloth. If you are going for a deep clean, remove the laces.

2 Dip a soft cloth in the polish or cream and start to work it gently into the shoe leather, making sure to cover the entire upper. The easiest way to apply it is by wrapping the cloth around your fingers. Replenish often. Leave to dry – about 15 minutes.

3 Brush the shoe vigorously, with the same circular motion you might use on your teeth – this helps make sure the polish is absorbed, and brings up the shine.

4 For extra shine, give it another going over with a (clean) soft cloth. If you are really serious, a little spit helps – the classic 'spit shine' involves multiple layers of polish and spit. Let it dry again, apply another layer of polish and repeat, endlessly.

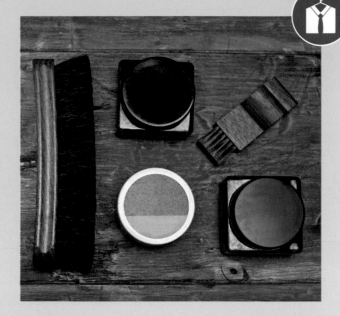

Cleaning suede shoes

Equipment

Suede brush, suede eraser block, kettle, washing-up sponge, suede protector.

1 Rub the shoes clean with the suede brush, brushing in one direction.

2 If stubborn stains won't come out first time, rub with a suede eraser block before brushing again.

3 Try the kettle trick. Put your hand in the shoe and hold it a safe distance over a steaming kettle (watch for scalding). Rub gently with the scouring side of a washing-up sponge before brushing the pile back up.

4 Apply protector spray – this will save you future cleaning hassle and help make the shoes waterproof.

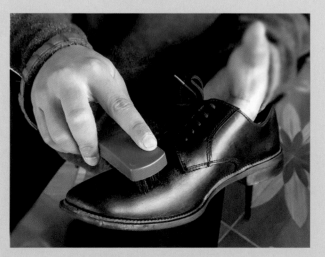

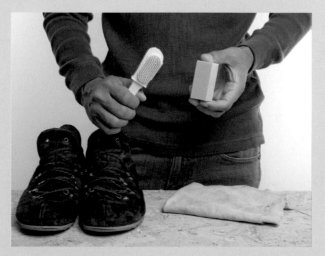

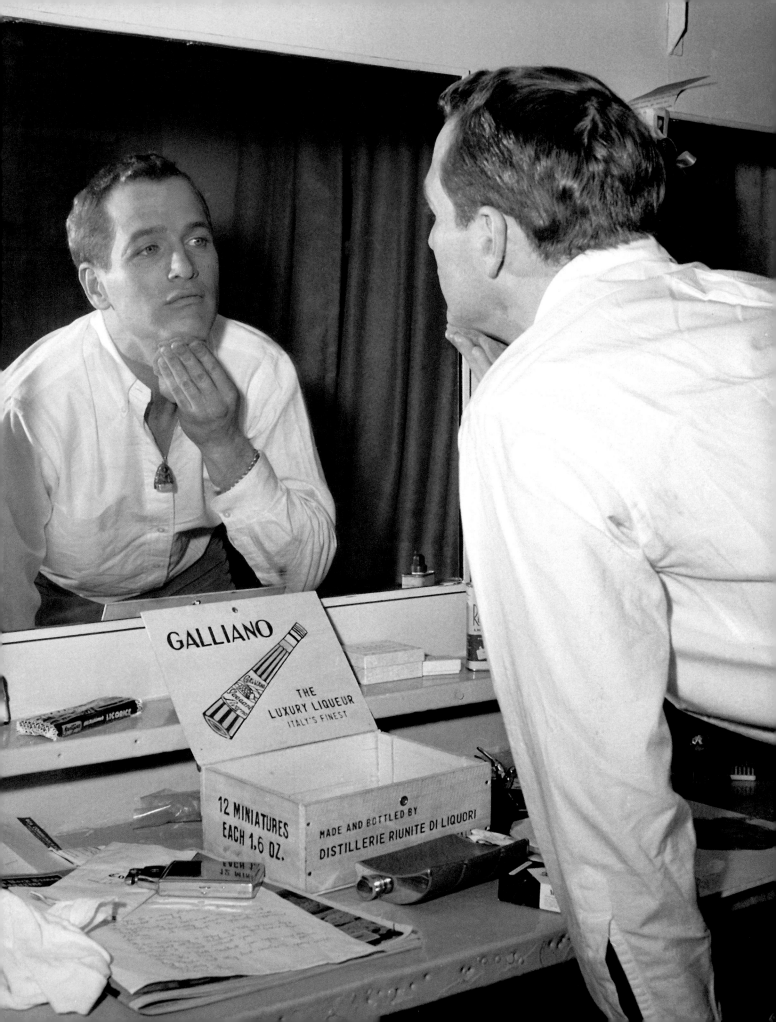

CHAPTER 4
GENERAL MANTENANCE

Man is a machine, and looking after it is your job. Cleaning, brushing, plucking, shaving, ensuring your person smells good and looks acceptable in swimwear, that both mind and body are ticking over nicely – all of that is on you. There is no denying it is a challenge. Happily, we live in an age in which a man can spend some time on himself without having to tolerate criticism (don't take it too far, though – vanity is never an attractive trait). Maintenance is now an accepted and expected part of being a man – pick up those nose-hair trimmers and get to work.

FITNESS

Twenty years ago, many men's idea of exercise was lifting a pint. Times have changed, and it's common for guys to spend the money their fathers would have passed on to the pub on protein shakes and Lycra shorts. Gym membership has exploded and the search for a lean, cut physique is now some people's main pursuit. Yet, despite the increased pressure to conform to an idealised, objectified idea of male good looks, obesity levels are at an all-time high.

Perfection vs reality

Some guys live in the gym, and some never leave the sofa. Both extremes are exactly that: extreme. There's nothing wrong with being fit – it is what every man, of every age, should be aiming for. But if your drive for that perfect body is seeing you work out every day, taking intense class after intense class, if you live in your gym, then you need to take a step back. The search for perfection can mask a deep unhappiness, and fitness does not mean abs you can grate cheese on. It means feeling strong, flexible and well. All of which can be achieved without setting foot in a gym.

The gym

The gym is a convenient place in which to get physical exercise, and has become an integral part of some guys' lives. Below are ways to go beyond it, to take your exercise in new and positive ways. If you do use the gym, make sure you are getting the most out of your time and effort.

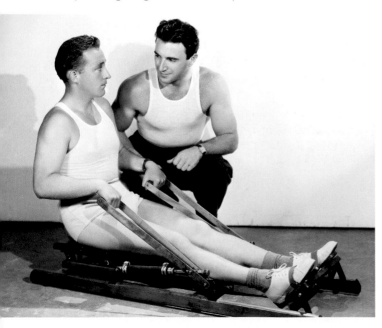

Take a look at what you are doing, and what your focus is. Is your priority a particular physical shape, or the ability to bench-press a certain weight? Physical fitness is about more than muscle mass, or attaining a certain physique. You need flexibility, core strength, good circulation and a healthy heart. That means mixing it up, going beyond the weights room and introducing cardio – good for your mental health and your heart. Yoga will help you maintain flexibility, and Pilates will help you keep your core strong, reducing the risk of back injuries and helping you stand up straight.

It may be an idea, if you don't know what you are doing, to get a personal trainer, a good one, and talk to them about what you want to achieve, what fitness means to you. Listen to their advice. At the very least, you should be walking into the gym with a plan for the session, including a decent warm-up/cool-down, a sensible ratio of weights to cardio and a big bottle of water.

The minimum for good health

The medical recommendation is that on a weekly basis adults should be doing either:

◆ at least 150 minutes of moderate aerobic activity (cycling, walking fast), along with strength exercises on the major muscle groups, or
◆ 75 minutes of vigorous aerobic activity (running, tennis) plus strength exercises as above, or
◆ a mixture of the two.

'Moderate' activity is the kind that makes your heart beat faster, but during which you can still hold a conversation – hiking, or riding a bike on the flat. 'Vigorous' is riding that bike up a hill, or breaking into a run. Muscle-strength exercising isn't just lifting weights – it could mean using your own body (sit-ups, press-ups), heavy gardening, yoga, Pilates. Intense activities such as circuit training, football, running, etc can count as being both aerobic and muscle strengthening.

Overdoing it

Recent research has shown that an addiction to high-intensity workouts may be very bad news. Combining a punishing workout routine with an already stressful work life can be as bad for the body as doing nothing at all. If your workouts result in repetitive strain injuries, or a weakened immune system, then it's time to slow down, mix it up. Give your muscles time to rest and recover after workouts. Remember, the body you can achieve depends on the body type you started with – not all guys were made to be bulky, or slim.

Cutting flab

If you want to lose weight, start with your diet. What you put in to your body will define how you look and feel as much as, (and in some cases more than) exercise. Without a balanced diet, featuring the right amounts of fruit and vegetables, proteins, carbs and fats, your fitness will always be limited. For weight loss, start by reducing starchy carbs, cutting down on sugar and breaking bad food habits in favour of something healthier.

Exercise-wise, you need to burn more calories than you consume. Lift weights, take cardio classes, run, but don't focus on one area alone. Work all the muscles in your body, not just those around your abs. Aerobic and strength exercises are going to burn the calories, but don't neglect those that bring flexibility and balance and give you a strong core, such as yoga and Pilates. Whatever regime you choose, the difference between success and failure is sticking with it – go for something you genuinely enjoy and will keep doing.

If you want to really enjoy fitness, try getting out of the gym. Of particular benefit are pursuits that get you

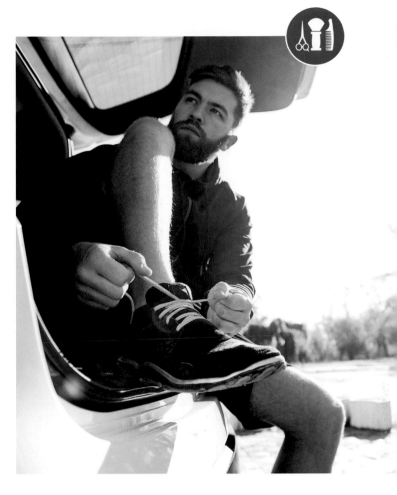

outside, where exercise is more interesting and stimulating; factors such as wind resistance and uneven ground mean you burn more calories; and fresh air and increased oxygen will help release serotonin, the brain chemical that makes you feel good. Also, unlike the gym, this is (mostly) free, and doesn't smell of other men's socks.

Getting out of the gym and away from the idea of shaping the perfect physique can be liberating, good for your body and mind, and if you're doing it with other people it's good for your social life too. All it takes is the nerve to look at the options around you and give it a go.

Using the everyday

If you are just getting into fitness, or want to incorporate it into a hectic life, it's OK to start small. Use what you've got. If you have a long bus ride to work, get off two stops early and walk the rest of the way. Go out and walk during lunch rather than just stay at your workstation. If you usually take the elevator, make mounting the stairs the norm. Desk jockeys should take regular screen breaks (at least 5 minutes every hour) and incorporate stretches to compensate for all that sitting time, and the bad posture it encourages. Add movement to your daily life as a regular habit and you will find the idea of taking on a more demanding exercise regime much less daunting.

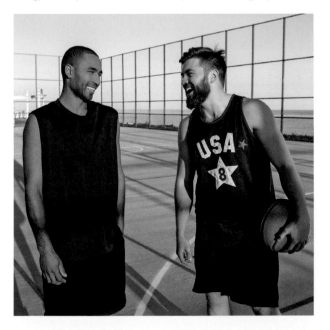

GET OUT OF THE GYM

Cycling

As the phenomenon of the Lycra Dad or MAMIL (middle-aged man in Lycra) proves, men love bikes. You get to lavish money on ridiculous kit, love interests will appreciate your shapely calves, and the endorphins that are produced from a demanding ride can send stress levels down and happiness up. Cycling saves you money, getting you there faster than walking and more cheaply than taking the bus, train or car. Folded into your daily life as part of your commute, it gets you fit by stealth, increasing your cardiovascular fitness and muscular strength, improving joint mobility and helping you shed fat and stress. If you are sensible with traffic and don't run red lights, your risk of injury is statistically relatively low.

You don't need to spend thousands, or wear Lycra, to get started. Get a decent bike second hand, making sure it is the right size for you and suits your plans for it. If you are broke, ask around friends and family – someone is bound to have one they never use. If you are sticking to roads, aim for a road bike, off-road adventuring requires a mountain bike, and a commuter bike will need to suit your work – eg folding up for the train. A good bike shop can give you advice on the best machine for your purposes, for free – but don't feel you have to buy new. Don't stint on safety features – helmet, lights – or a lock. If you find yourself getting serious, join a club – it will motivate you, help you kick it up a gear and bring in a social element.

Running

Running is the oldest form of exercise, if you don't count swinging through the trees, or sex. It removes excess adrenaline and stress, shifts body fat, burns calories, and lifts your mood and fitness levels. And all you need to start is a decent pair of shoes and a sense of determination.

Start by walking. Really. If you are new to this sort of exercise, starting at a sprint will destroy you, ending the habit before it has begun. Instead, set yourself a training schedule, buy some running shoes and start with a brisk walk every day. Once your heart is pumping, incorporate short stretches of running. As you get into it, and your legs and lungs adapt to the new challenge, change the ratio in favour of running – but be sure to incorporate a decent warm-up and cool-down, walking and stretching.

Posture is important – keep your head up, your shoulders relaxed, and your back straight. If motivation is proving difficult, try incorporating music or a running partner, or use an app/wearable tech to monitor your progress. Running clubs are everywhere, as are informal drop-in weekly runs.

Triathlons

Triathlon combines swimming, running and cycling, and delivers the health benefits of each. If you're already fit, and thrive on a challenge, then it may be for you. If you are unfit, and looking for a challenge to motivate you, then look at taking on a distance or format suited to your level –

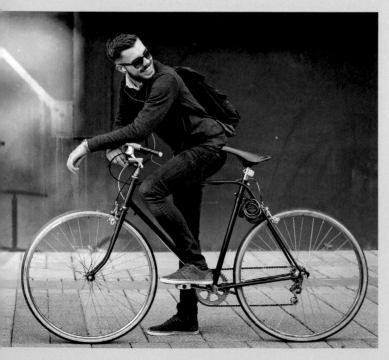

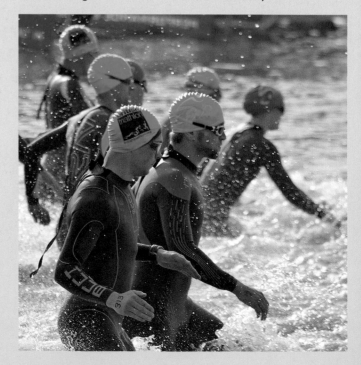

there are easier ways to get fit than the Olympic distances, the cardio equivalent of climbing Everest. For beginners the 'supersprint' triathlon incorporates a 400m swim, a 10km bike ride and a 5km run. If you want more of a challenge, the 'sprint distance' race breaks down as 750m, 20km, 10km. Whichever you choose, the key will be a well-planned training regime. Equipment-wise, you will need a swimming costume or wetsuit and a bike/helmet.

Surfing

Surfing is the true sport of kings, an intense and (mostly) fun workout that will leave you energised and stoked. The paddling brings cardiovascular fitness and shoulder/back strength, while riding and balancing on the board builds core and leg strength. Stress is entirely stripped away. You may never be Kelly Slater, but the best surfer in the water is the one having the most fun.

The best way to learn to surf is to combine it with a holiday. Book yourself a week somewhere with accommodation, equipment and lessons provided. By day three you will be weeping with tiredness, aching in places you didn't know existed, but by day seven you will be up and riding. It is possible to teach yourself to surf, but the odds are you will develop bad habits (like popping up to your knees first). If you are determined, get yourself a big, floaty board and play around in the white water until you know what you are doing. Paddle hard to catch a wave, push your chest up off the board to accelerate into it, and pop up quickly – back foot at right angles to the board, front foot at a 45-degree angle. Learn surfing etiquette – don't go for a wave someone is already on.

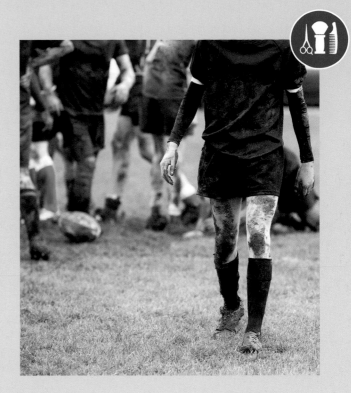

Team sports

Joining a team will get you fit without you noticing, apart from post-match aches and pains. Football/soccer, rugby, basketball, baseball, cricket – all will burn calories, boost fitness levels, and build endurance, while the competitive structure and camaraderie will make it considerably more fun than working out alone.

Don't be put off by a relative lack of skill or fitness. Almost every ball sport will have a variety of levels, open to beginners. Football/soccer requires only a ball, a park and a friend, and there is an enormous range of leagues and teams for all abilities and ages. Touch rugby – no tackling, so no lost teeth – can be played with a handful of willing friends, or join a team to commit to training and building your strength and stamina. Cricket is traditionally played on a field, with teams of 11 – but new, accessible, indoor versions are increasingly popular.

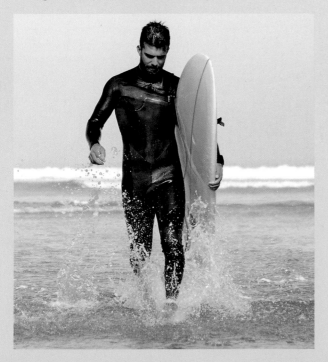

'If you always put limits on everything you do, physical or anything else, it will spread into your life. There are no limits. There are only plateaus, and you must not stay there, you must go beyond them'
Bruce Lee

THE HEALTHY MAN

Taking your health and fitness seriously relies on you learning to listen to your body and being sensitive to its needs. A man has to care for and monitor himself – do not ignore the blinking lights that warn of trouble ahead. Managing your health means getting used to what you are like when everything is working well, and recognising the signs that suggest you aren't. It also means knowing when to seek help – which is the bit most men struggle with…

When to see a doctor

Many men put up with ailments that could be easily treated, living with low-level pain and discomfort as if this is inevitable. According to the statistics, men visit the doctor half as often as women, preferring instead to lick their wounds in private, or relying on Dr Google. If something is bothering you, causing you to worry, don't be shy of seeing your GP. No matter how embarrassing or ridiculous the complaint, it is guaranteed they will have seen worse and will not laugh. If there is an issue that is niggling you but it doesn't seem significant enough for the doctor, see a chemist – they can do much more than recommend products.

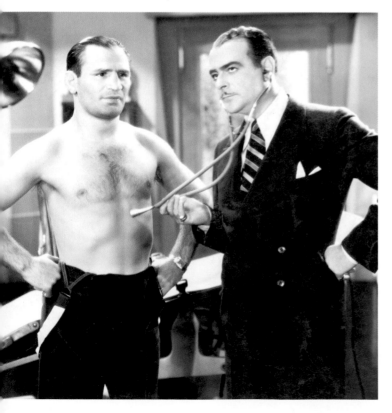

Common manly malfunctions

Although we are more likely to think of ourselves as infallible, men are just as prone to getting ill as the fairer sex, and it's wise to recognise this. More often than not minor illnesses are just that – minor – and are best treated with a course of bed rest, self-pity, lots of fluids and a line-up of TV box sets. There will be other times when you really should visit the doctor or seek other medical help. The following is intended as a guide to help you work out which scenario you are experiencing, but if in doubt do err on the side of caution and ask an expert – better safe than sorry.

Manflu

Manflu is a disparaging phrase for any cold, flu or mystery virus that wipes a chap out, making him feel useless and tired and likely to whine loudly about it to an unsympathetic partner. Some men soldier on through such viruses, slogging into work to infect their colleagues, prolonging the illness so that they can continue to claim their 'no sick days' medal. Don't be this man. If you feel wretched, take it easy. Drink fluids, rest, watch daytime TV, wait for it to pass. If it doesn't, get to a doctor.

Food poisoning

You can't live an interesting culinary life without risking a bout of food poisoning – an unwitting exposure to bacteria such as salmonella or E. coli. Common culprits include bad shellfish and poor kitchen hygiene. You will know it was something you ate if the illness kicks in a few hours after eating, leading to vomiting, diarrhoea, weakness, chills and aches, though it can take up to 48 hours, or even in some cases several weeks, to make itself apparent. If you are caught, there isn't much to be done but ride it out, staying hydrated.

When you feel able to take food again, stick to BRAT – bananas, rice, (grated or puréed) apple, dry toast – until you feel well enough to start to eat normally again, usually

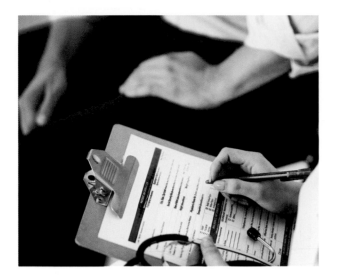

24–48 hours. To start with, avoid greasy, spicy foods and alcohol since these can upset a delicate stomach. Try to think of it as a detox. It may also be an idea to buy some probiotics to take afterwards in order to replenish the bacteria in your gut, which will have been seriously disrupted by the event.

Athlete's foot

Athlete's foot is a nasty fungal rash that appears between the toes – often brought on by a failure to keep your feet clean/dry. If you notice itchy, red skin, treat it ASAP with a cream or spray from the chemist, and revise your foot-hygiene routine, making sure you always dry them thoroughly and wear clean cotton socks. It is infectious, so avoid sharing towels and don't walk around barefoot in the gym.

Depression

By far the saddest statistic in men's health is depression. Women are more likely to experience it, but men are more likely to die from it – probably because they don't seek help.

Depression is an illness, and your mental health is just as important as your physical health. The next section will give you some ideas on managing yours, but if you feel trapped in extreme sadness, see your GP. Depression is treatable, and becoming well again starts from the moment you ask for help.

Accidents

Men experience higher rates of death from unintentional injury, often from the wide range of exciting and stupid things we are statistically more likely to do – eg mucking about with fireworks. We are also far more likely to die behind the wheel and through an occupational injury. The only thing these deaths and injuries have in common is that they are, for the most part, eminently avoidable. Follow Health and Safety rules, particularly when you've been drinking alcohol, and look before you leap, both literally and figuratively.

HOW TO
STAND UP STRAIGHT

If you can make one positive change to your life, right now, make it this: stand up straight. Good posture improves your looks and your health, relieves back pain, and makes you appear more attractive and feel more confident. The technology of our age doesn't help – we are used to crouching over laptops, cradling phones in our neck, slumping at a desk.

You can train yourself to have good posture – the aim is to hold your body in a position while standing (or sitting) in which you place less strain on your muscles. It may feel odd at first, but when you make a conscious habit of correcting yourself it will eventually become second nature.

Stand up, in your natural position, feet shoulder-width apart, toes pointing forwards. Now picture someone grabbing a hair at the top of your head and pulling it up. Let it raise you up, keeping your shoulders relaxed. Engage your core muscles, pulling in your abdomen, keeping your weight evenly balanced on both feet. Let your arms hang, and try to avoid slumping into your lower back, locking your knees or sticking out your bottom. This is what good posture feels like. I know, weird, but you look taller already.

'You are allowed to feel messed up and inside out. It doesn't mean you're defective – it just means you're human'
David Mitchell

HOW TO
PROTECT THE FAMILY JEWELS

Your balls are a significant part of your package. However, most men neglect them in favour of their more prominent neighbour, thinking of them only when there is a risk they might get kicked.

Ball care can be learned. Get in the habit of keeping them cool with comfortable underwear and be aware that a source of heat, such as a laptop or mobile/cell phone can harm your sperm. Use a table for hardware and use a different pocket for your phone. As noted below, testicular cancer is more treatable when caught early. Learning how to check your family jewels may save your life. See below.

BTW it is relatively common for men to think their balls are weird, because balls are weird. The odds are that yours are no more unusual than anyone else's, but again, if in doubt, ask a GP. He or she has seen it all before.

Prostate cancer

Your prostate is a gland you probably take for granted, situated just below the bladder, producing some of the fluid in semen. Prostate cancer is a common cancer for men. An enlarged prostate can make it hard to pee, or cause a burning sensation, which may be cancer or something much less alarming. See the GP, to be on the safe side.

Testicular cancer

The most common form of cancer in young men is testicular. Treatment is much more effective when the cancer is caught early. Get used to checking your balls regularly, so you know what 'different' feels like. To do so, hold the penis out of the way and check the testicles one at a time. Hold each between thumb and fingers and roll it gently. You are looking for any solid lumps or smooth, round bumps, or anything else that does not feel right – like a change in the size, shape or hardness. When you get to know them as you should, this will feel more natural and slightly less weird. Now wash your hands. If in doubt, get them checked out.

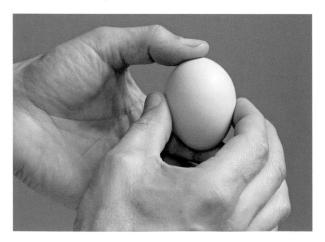

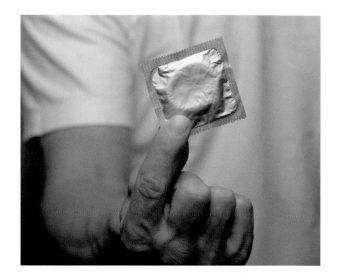

STIs

Most sexually active men are likely to have some sort of brush with a sexually transmitted disease (STD) or infection (STI) at some point. If you feel burning, redness or itching, or see discharge down below, don't panic. Get yourself to the GP, or to a sexual health/genitourinary medicine (GUM) clinic ASAP. An early diagnosis can put your mind at rest if it is something simple, and help save your health if it is something more serious. Currently common STD/STIs include:

- chlamydia: pain/burning while peeing, cloudy discharge, tender testicles
- genital warts: probably painless small bumps/skin changes around your genitals or anus. Common, and can be passed on without penetration.
- genital herpes: small, painful blisters around the penis, itchy or tingly
- gonorrhoea: a bacterial infection that may or may not produce any symptoms. A burning sensation while peeing, a discharge – white, yellow, or green – from the tip of the penis, tender or painful testicles.
- syphilis: serious bacterial infection, beginning with a painless but highly infectious sore on the genitals or mouth. Secondary signs include a rash, flu-like symptoms and hair loss.
- HIV: a virus that attacks the immune system, weakening it. Early symptoms may include a flu-like illness with a fever, sore throat or rash. Get yourself tested.
- crabs: pubic lice. Itching and signs of eggs or lice on your pubes. Don't worry, you won't have to shave them.
- scabies: tiny mites. Look for intense itching in your genitals, on hands, under arms. A rash may be possible.

By the way, if you were thinking of not wearing a condom, ever, read the above list again.

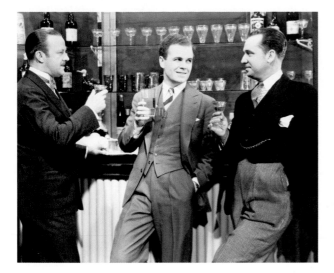

HOW TO
AVOID HANGOVERS

Q: What's the best thing for a hangover?
A: Drinking heavily the night before.

If you're living with a hangover, humour is not going to help. But it is coming your way anyway, along with a total lack of sympathy. Because it doesn't matter how utterly rotten you feel – you brought this on yourself. The best strategy is never letting it happen again. Know when to say no. If you don't feel like getting drunk, don't agree to a sixth beer or to tequila (ever). Alternate drinks with water, order halves instead of pints, sit out the occasional round, and stick to one type of alcohol. Drink a pint of water when you get home, and keep another by the bed.

If you didn't take that advice, and you are imagining there is a fantastic recipe that will cure your raging hangover, dream on. Man has searched for this cure since time immemorial, and has only come up with Alka-Seltzer. Rehydrate with something that contains electrolytes (coconut water, rehydration tablets in water, sports drink), take paracetamol, and if you can face it, eat breakfast.

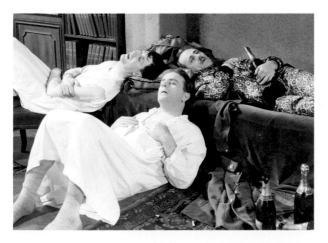

HOW TO
RECOGNISE ALCOHOL ADDICTION

For some, alcohol may come across as man's best friend, but there can come a point when it becomes his mortal enemy. Learning to tell the difference is the key to enjoying it safely, in moderation. If you do choose to drink, watch for the warning signs of addiction:

◆ being unable to control when, or how much, you drink
◆ building up a tolerance that means you need more alcohol to feel the effect
◆ storing alcohol in unusual places
◆ having to drink to feel normal
◆ drinking alone, or in secret
◆ being irritable if you can't drink when you want to
◆ continuing to drink, even when you know it has had a negative effect on your life or relationships
◆ experiencing blackouts
◆ feeling physical withdrawal symptoms – nausea, sweating, shaking, etc.

If you recognise those reactions, in you or someone close to you, there may be a problem. Help is available, if you need it – for addressing it in someone else, or facing it in yourself.

Excessive drinking may be a problem, even if it isn't (yet) alcoholism. Look honestly at how much you drink in an average week. If it is regularly over the recommendations of the experts (currently 14 units per week for men, which is about 6 pints of weakish beer) you may need to cut down.

Dealing with addiction

Addiction is not only about alcohol – apparently one in three men are addicted to something. People can become dependent on drugs (legal and otherwise) gambling, sex, pornography, gaming ... pretty much anything that may be enjoyable in small doses is potentially addictive. If there is regular behaviour you are finding difficult to stop, or cut down on, which is causing problems in other areas of your life, dominating your thoughts, making you feel like you are not in control, or causing withdrawal feelings, you may have a problem.

You are not alone. Whatever the addiction, there is a community of people who have been through it and come out the other side, so if you recognise this pattern, reach out – to AA, NA, the National Gambling Helpline, your GP, a counsellor, a friend.

HOW TO
COPE IN MEDICAL EMERGENCIES

In emergency situations, your first job is to stay calm. Breathe. You are an adult man. You've got this. If in doubt, and you believe this is serious, call an ambulance. Better to err on the side of caution; the paramedic team are not going to give you a hard time if they turn up and find that everyone is OK.

Fainting/dizziness
While you wait for medical help, check the patient's alertness – can they answer a question? If they are conscious, keep them comfortable – if it's hot, move them into the shade, get them a drink. If they are unconscious but breathing, move them into the recovery position. If they aren't breathing, start cardiopulmonary resuscitation (CPR).

Chest pain
There are lots of reasons why someone might have chest pain but the safest assumption is that it's a heart attack. Call the emergency services, then check airways and breathing and pulse. If they are not breathing, try CPR.

Bleeding
Most cuts aren't going to cause you or anyone else to bleed to death. However, if blood is gushing or you are otherwise worried, call an ambulance. If you have cut a tendon, or may need stitches, if you can't stop the bleeding, if you can't move the affected area, if there's a lot of damage or a risk of infection (or you were bitten) get medical attention, ASAP.

CPR
Cardiopulmonary resuscitation is what you've seen people on TV do to keep someone alive until the medics arrive. You can pick up this skill on a first-aid course, along with rescue breaths, but if you find yourself in a situation where it might help, it is generally better to attempt chest compressions than to do nothing. You are trying to preserve brain activity and prevent tissue damage, until someone with the right equipment can get circulation and breathing back again.

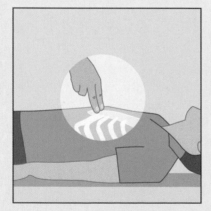

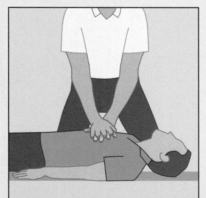

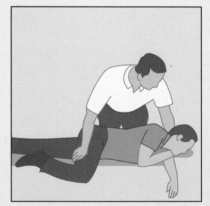

1 Find the breastbone in the centre of the patient's chest, then put the heel of your hand on top. Put the other hand on top and lock the fingers together.

2 Position yourself on top, with your shoulders over your hands. Use your body weight to push down hard on the chest, by about 5cm/2in. Release, let the chest rise up, and repeat at a rate of 100 to 120 times per minute.

3 Continue for as long as you can or until help arrives. If the patient begins to take breaths, move them into the recovery position, on their side, top leg bent.

For smaller cuts, apply direct pressure to the site of the cut with a clean, dry material – eg a towel – for several minutes. If the cut is on your arm, holding it up above your head will reduce the flow. If it is on lower limbs, lie down and put the affected area in the air.

Once the bleeding has stopped, clean the wound – wash and dry your hands, then run the cut under clean running tap water. Pat dry and apply a sterile dressing or adhesive bandage. If this is a big one, you may need stitches.

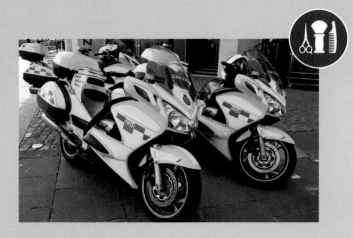

Burns

Immediately cool the burn under cool running water for 20 minutes. Don't use ice or anything very cold, since this can cause frostbite on already damaged skin, and don't use anything greasy, such as creams or butter.

If anything is stuck to the skin, don't attempt to move it. Burns can be covered with clingfilm or a clean plastic bag. Keep it clean and don't attempt to burst any blisters.

For serious burns, you will need medical attention immediately. 'Serious' includes:

◆ any chemical/electrical burns
◆ large (bigger than your hand) or deep burns
◆ any burns that cause white or charred skin
◆ burns that cause blisters in sensitive areas (face, arms, legs, feet, genitals, hands).

Choking

If a person at the next table is choking, someone will need to perform the Heimlich Manoeuvre. They won't be able to tell you they need help – if they are coughing, there is still air movement, so hold off – if they go quiet/start turning red, move quickly, there may be only a few minutes to save a life. You can also perform the Heimlich Manoeuvre on yourself, by pressing the abdomen sharply, in the same place, on to a chair, or with the same hand thrust.

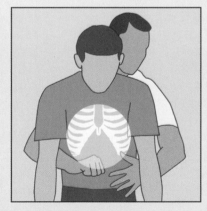

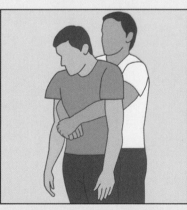

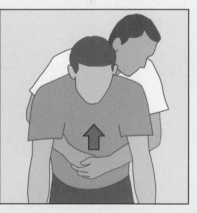

1 Stand behind the person choking, with your legs separated for balance. Reach around and grab your hands together, making a fist with your dominant hand, just above their belly button and below the breastbone.

2 Tuck your thumb out of the way. Pull inwards and then upwards, pressing into the abdomen with quick thrusts. Act as if you are trying to lift the person off their feet.

3 Keep up the series of thrusts until whatever is in there is expelled. Use a gentler force on a child. If the choking person falls unconscious, stop the manoeuvre.

MENTAL HEALTH

Suicide is the biggest killer of men under the age of 45 in the UK. In one recent year, 75% of all UK suicides were male. Take a moment to reflect on that statistic and what it says about the risks that face us. Not sharks, not zombies, not terrorist attacks, but our own mental health. We don't face more stress or depression than women – but we are far more likely to die from it.

Some men believe that asking for help or talking about troubles is a sign of weakness and indicates a loss of control. Somewhere along the line they learn that men are supposed to be strong, resolute despite everything life chucks at them. Except that for most of us, it doesn't work like that. There will be periods when we are at a low ebb, because of things that have happened to us or a mood we can't shift. At that point, we are more vulnerable because, unlike many women, we don't feel right talking about it, or telling someone – anyone – when it has become more than we can bear.

Depression

Real depression is hugely common, and little understood. It is easy to sink into it unawares, and hard to say when a low mood has given way to something darker, and harder to escape. It is more than temporary sadness – this is a state you can't pull yourself out of. It's as real as any physical condition, and it takes time and help to recover from it.

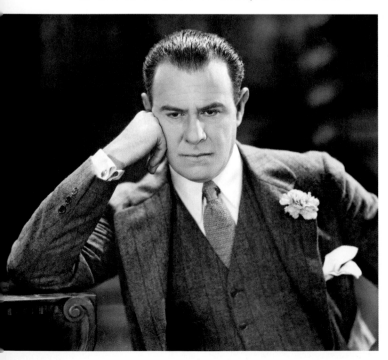

The charity CALM (the Campaign Against Living Miserably) describes some of the signs: low confidence; feeling worthless or guilty; unable to enjoy life. We may be irritable, snappy, take to drugs or drink to manage; experience deep anxiety, negative thoughts, low energy; or feel unable to get to sleep or to wake up, trapped, unable to reach out. Severe depression may be all of the above, and more. CALM describe three symptoms:

◆ hating or disliking yourself
◆ hating the world around you and wanting to escape it
◆ seeing little hope or future for yourself.

If that sounds familiar, don't suffer in silence. You can recover from depression, but it starts with accepting it is happening – and asking for help. This can come in many forms – treatment available via your GP can include counselling, meditation, exercise programmes, cognitive behavioural therapy (CBT), or anti-depressants. Help via your friends may vary – sometimes people think they should offer solutions, when all you may need is a sympathetic ear, so if you choose to share, do so with someone you feel will really listen. There are Internet forums and helplines that will enable you to realise you are not alone. Talking to a professional can help you to understand what you're going through, get some perspective, and change unhealthy patterns.

Stress and anxiety

Work, exams, love, money – lots of very real factors can make you feel like you are under threat. In small doses, anxiety can help you stay on top of things – it is the normal, biological response to danger. When it starts to take over, though, it can overwhelm you, bringing both physical symptoms and a sense of panic. If you feel that sense of threat all the time, your anxiety may have become a problem. A lot of mental health is about feeling a sense of security. When men have experienced difficult childhoods, they may be more vulnerable to anxiety issues.

It's easy to take refuge in alcohol and drugs – legal and otherwise. Such measures can deal with the short-term stress, but they don't solve what's underneath it. You need to get to the source of the problem and try to make sense of where this is coming from…

Stress control

Talking is a good start. Some people find keeping a diary helps them to understand what they are experiencing. Anything that takes you away from focusing on problems is a good thing – sports, exercise, gardening, a long walk, listening to music, or an exercise class with an emphasis on breathing – yoga, Pilates. Be outside. If your life is lived at a desk and on a commute, take time off to go for a walk, preferably in a natural environment. Technology can add to stress levels in busy, connected lives, particularly the constant presence of social media. Take a regular digital detox, turning off your phone for an evening. Live in the analogue world for a bit, with a book, a bath, a record, a real-world conversation.

Meditation

Meditation can help stress control and with managing the physical symptoms of anxiety, encouraging you to relax and find balance, and to let go of the things you can't control. Quieting your thoughts can help you understand your feelings. Learning to meditate is easier than you might think. There are many techniques, which can be learned in the same way as physical exercise. It helps to join a class, but there is no reason why you can't get started on your own – there are good free apps to help, or just begin.

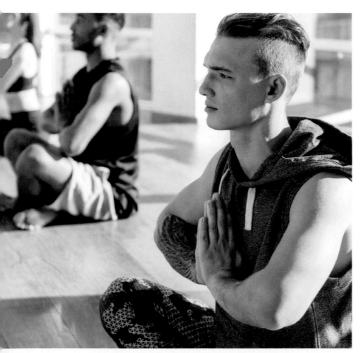

Happiness

Much of what is in our lives is beyond our control. Nevertheless it is open to us to take charge of our approach, to make a deliberate and mindful decision to aim for a happier life. That decision can help us make better choices about life, love and work. The charity Action for Happiness have identified 10 keys that consistently deliver more happiness to most people. If you are struggling to find happiness, the checklist is a good place to start:

- do things for others
- connect with people
- take care of your body
- live life mindfully
- keep learning new things
- have goals to look forward to
- find ways to bounce back
- look for what's good
- be comfortable with who you are
- be part of something bigger.

Sit or lie comfortably, in a safe place. Close your eyes. Don't aim to control your breathing, just let it happen. Start to pay attention to how you breathe and the effect it has on your body. This is concentration meditation, where you will focus on one thing – in this case, your breath. As you feel your attention wandering, bring it back to your breathing, Start with a few minutes at a time, and then try longer – you'll find with practice you are able to concentrate for longer periods.

Breathing exercises for panic

If you have ever experienced a panic attack, you'll know how terrifying it can be. The symptoms are real, and feel genuinely life threatening. Breathing exercises can help get you through stressful times. Concentrate on your breathing. Breathe in deeply, through your nose. Try to take the breath deep into you and, placing your hands on your stomach, feel it expand as the breath enters. Relax your shoulders. Exhale slowly through your mouth. Repeat, releasing tension and anxiety with the exhale.

ESSENTIAL MANTENANCE

Some aspects of a man's person require more attention than others – mostly those from the neck up, since that is where the majority of people will be looking. In particular, if you sport any kind of beard, you'll need to take care of it. It's as much a question of comfort as style – poorly maintained facial hair can look and feel like a mess.

Likewise, a man needs to exercise some control over every hair that sprouts from his person. Most importantly of all, he has to manage how he smells – the invisible but powerful force that can wreck his chances or make his night.

There is a fine balance to be struck, however. On the one hand, you need to look after yourself, and make sure you are well turned out. On the other, a guy who spends a fortune on cosmetics and takes two hours to get ready, is not most people's idea of a confident, attractive man. Aim for the middle ground. Start by establishing a bathroom routine with an emphasis on low effort.

Facial care

The men's cosmetic industry is worth a fortune, which may help explain why magazines and online advertising will suggest you need a very expensive tub of cream or else your face will fall off. It won't. You can get by on three good quality basic products.

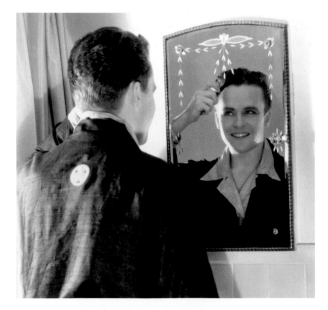

A foaming cleanser

You need something that cleans the face, without the harsh drying qualities of a bar of soap. Choose a product that is suitable for your skin type, ideally non-fragranced. It doesn't have to be for men – you may find a cleanser marketed at women works for you. Clean gently first thing in the morning and last thing at night: open the pores first with a splash of warm water, then apply. Rinse off the product completely (a flannel helps) and finish with a splash of cool water to close the pores. Pat dry, and follow up with a moisturiser.

Moisturiser

This is the most important item in your bathroom cupboard. Life is dirty and hard, and the skin on your face is delicate. Protect it with a moisturiser that suits your skin type. Moisturise in the morning and at night. Don't overdo it – a little goes a long way. Using a moisturiser with UV protection in the morning is a good idea.

Scrub

Regular exfoliation helps to remove dead skin and other gunk, unblocking the pores and saving you from blackheads etc. Depending on the sensitivity of your skin, this might be a weekly or bi-weekly routine – men with oilier skin may find it helps guard against spots. A scrub is handled in the same way as a cleanser (above), but is easiest used in the shower.

Extras

If you are serious about this then don't let me stop you investing in miracle products designed to make you look 21 forever. Some of these products may even work. However, bear in mind that vanity is unattractive and age is inevitable. Eye cream can conceal the effects of a wild/sleepless night by shrinking the bags a little. An occasional clay mask is a good way of deep-cleaning – as is a professional facial. Some men with oily skin use toner in between the wash and moisturiser.

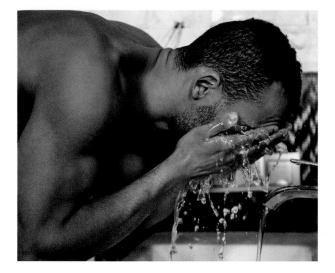

Dealing with spots

First rule of dealing with spots: leave them alone. Do not poke, squeeze or otherwise muck around with acne – it will make it worse and may leave scars. Despite what we were told, spots do not magically disappear when you turn 18. Or 21. Or 35. The good news is they are likely to fade into the background as you get older, bar the occasional flare-up. There are plenty of over-the-counter acne treatments – including face washes containing benzoyl peroxide. If yours is bad and not getting better, talk to the doctor – there are other options.

Shaving with spots is an undeniable pain. Use a gentle anti-bacterial cleanser first, and a good shaving cream or oil to help the razor along – clear products will help you shave around the spots. If you can't avoid shaving over them, use very light pressure and always go with the direction of hair growth. A little stubble is preferable to skin trauma.

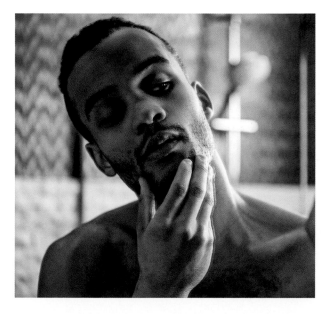

Skin types

Men, if you believe cosmetics companies, have different types of facial skin, depending on how sensitive, dry or oily it is. Diagnosing yours can help save you time in the skin-product aisle.

Normal: If you don't know what you are, but nothing seems wrong, then this is probably you. Lucky man. Follow the basic regime.

Dry: If your skin is dry, dull, rough to the touch, with red patches and not very elastic, this is you. Lines may appear more visible and your skin can crack or become irritated easily. Take shorter showers, use the mildest soaps and cleansers, and slap on a rich moisturiser, as often as needed.

Oily: You may have a shiny or dull complexion, enlarged pores, or suffer from regular outbreaks of spots and blackheads. The excess oil can come from your hormones, from stress, or from the awesome combination of the two we call puberty. Don't over-wash your skin, which may cause even more excess oil – use a gentle cleanser and consider a toner. Look for products that won't block your pores.

Combination: In some areas your skin is fine, but in others you may be either dry or oily. Often this is in the 'T-zone' around your nose, forehead and chin – if you have open pores there, blackheads or shiny skin, this is you. Adopt a sensible middle ground, paying special attention to the needs of the problem areas.

Sensitive: Your skin is easily irritated, flaring up with redness, dryness and itchiness. It could be you are sensitive to certain triggers – and these can include skin products. Keep it simple and use as few, always unscented, and gentle products as you can until you have worked out what causes the outbreaks.

Everyman: Whatever your skin type, the following guidelines apply:

◆ Wearing sunscreen and avoiding too much direct sunlight is best for your skin. A tan looks good, but wrinkles and skin cancer don't.
◆ Stay hydrated. Drink plenty of water.
◆ Wash your skin properly at least once a day.
◆ Moisturise at least once a day.

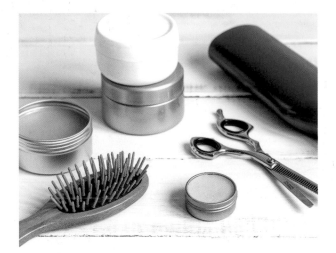

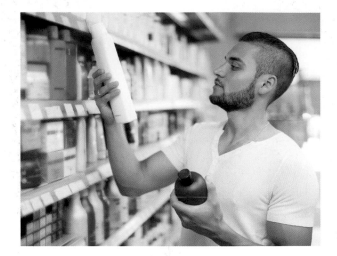

Hair care

If you want to confuse a man, take him to the haircare aisle and leave him there. Everything is packaged and marketed at people who know what kind of hair they have – yet most men would struggle to answer this question with anything other than 'yes'. Here are a few tips that will help you navigate your way through the countless products and work out what you really need.

Shampoo/conditioner

The first thing to ask yourself is whether or not you have dandruff. If you don't know, wear a black top and stand under a UV light – or ask someone. If you do, you'll need a shampoo that will deal with it (also, don't brush your hair while wearing dark clothes). Ditto greasy hair – again, you will know if this is what your hair tends towards. Dry hair is recognisable by its thick, dull qualities and will benefit from something with a bit of shine/moisturiser, as will tight curls. Fine, or thinning hair will look its best with a product that adds volume. If none of this sounds familiar, your hair is probably 'normal'.

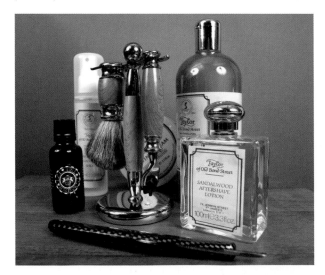

If in doubt, go for the product containing the least amount of chemical additions and the picture of the alpine meadow or similar on the front. Health-food stores are a good place to buy simple, natural beauty products. Avoid ones with a strong, chemical smell – you want all your fragrance to be chosen by you, not the laboratory.

Shampoo your hair two to three times a week, maximum, unless you do a lot of sport or have very oily hair – more will strip your hair of protective oils. Between shampoos, washing your hair with water will keep grease levels down.

Condition once a week – more can cause a build-up. Avoid scalding heat – cooler water is less damaging. Hair is vulnerable when it is wet, so don't treat it roughly with a towel or brush – letting it dry naturally keeps it strong.

Styling products

Depending on your style and hair type, you will probably need some sort of hair product to keep your follicles in check. The best product is the one recommended by your barber/hairdresser – ask their advice.

There are a huge number of styling products, from super-light gels to gunky pomades. If you have a short style, all you may want is a light oil or wax for gloss. Gels are light, and wash/brush out easily – but they can flake, and feel unpleasant on the skin. Curly and thick hair will appreciate the holding power of old-school pomade. It can be murder to wash out, though, so use it sparingly. Remember to think not only about how you look but how someone would feel running their hand through your locks.

Apply the product on damp hair and comb or brush through. A military-style bristle brush can give a sharp, slick finish and men with curly/tangled hair should use a brush or comb with wider teeth to avoid frizzing. Don't use a hair dryer every day – the heat is damaging, especially on thinning or fine hair. Blow against the direction of growth for volume, or with it for a flat, controlled look.

GREY AND RECEDING HAIR

Dealing with greying hair

Just as some men lose their hair prematurely, some lose their colour sooner than expected. As with baldness, the difference between looking good and looking rueful is attitude. Accept it is happening, and don't take drastic steps to hide it. Male hair dyes are available to remove the grey discreetly, but the truth is that they can make it look a little … fake. If you are set on getting it dyed, it is worth visiting a salon and letting the pros do it.

Greying hair tends to be wiry and coarse, so shorter haircuts often look best – and are easier to control. Grey can also look a little dull and yellow; bring some shine to proceedings by using a conditioner designed for silvery hair. Yes, it is the man's equivalent of the blue rinse, but it works. Matte products are recommended for silver foxes, because oily waxes may give it a yellowish tinge.

Dealing with receding hair

It is an unhappy fact of life that many men will lose their hair. How extreme you want to be in the face of hair loss will be informed by your attitude to it. Remember that what is sexy is confidence – a man who is happy with himself and comfortable in his skin. If he is bitter, insecure or pretending the baldness isn't happening, that is going to be more difficult.

Don't let it mess you up. The nuclear option is always available: get your hair cropped short. When you get over the shock of the sight of your scalp, you may be surprised by how good this looks on you.

If you decide to fight against the progress of male-pattern baldness, you need to take great care of

what you've got. Wash and style your hair gently and carefully. Take vitamin and mineral supplements – this won't bring back lost hair, but it'll help with what's still there. Use products designed to maximise volume. Talk to your hairdresser about a strategy to use what you have, and draw attention away from thinning areas. Over-the-counter medications are available to promote hair growth and help prevent future loss. As for hair-transplant technology, the bald truth is that the most expensive treatments in the world still make you look like you've had a hair transplant: not a good look.

Receding: dos and don'ts

Don't: Hide it under a hat. This just makes people wonder what's under there.

Don't: Attempt a comb-over.

Don't: Wear a toupee.

Do: Be down with your own bad bald self.

Do: Keep your scalp clean and moisturised – use a matte finishing product to avoid scalp gleam.

Do: Take advice from your hairdresser – and if you think your baldness may be related to medication or stress, see your doctor.

Do: Go for a short hairstyle.

Do: Consider facial hair.

Do: Protect your head from the sun with cream and wear a hat.

⌄ Silver hair can look sophisticated and mature – let it work for you.

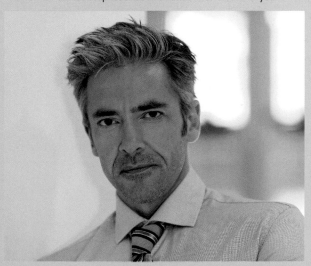

⌄ The world is full of attractive men with next to no hair on their heads.

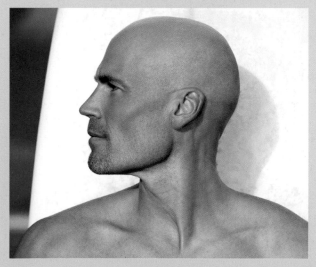

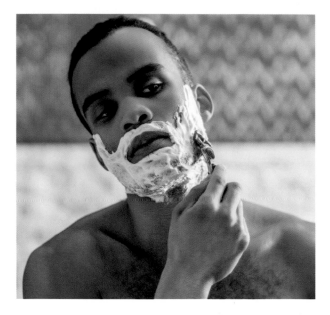

The art of shaving

If anything in a man's life is likely to lead to avoidable blood, sweat and tears, it is his razor blade. Or worse, his lady-friend's heavily used lady-bic, because guess who forgot to buy new blades? The key to shaving success is in the preparation, the care and the equipment. It is also true that it gets easier as you get to know your face. By the time you are 50, you'll be wielding a straight razor like a pro … though there may be a few nicks along the way.

Preparation

Always shave, if you can, after a hot shower or bath. The heat will soften the hairs, meaning you will be able to slice through them like a Samurai powering through warm butter. The absolute ideal is to shave in the shower – but you will need a fog-proof mirror for that. A shave after a Turkish bath or steam is also a pleasure, but if you can't manage that, apply a hot flannel for a minute or two before starting. At the very least, give yourself a good face wash and/or exfoliate before reaching for the razor. Never, ever, shave dry.

How often?

How regularly you shave depends on your face and your workplace. If the former is sensitive and the latter is laid-back, every two to three days is fine. Otherwise, just give yourself the weekend off.

Equipment

This is one area where going budget will hurt. Life is too short to use cheap disposable razors. If you are not yet a confident shaver, you can't go wrong with a cartridge blade. They are irritatingly expensive, but they go for five or so shaves before they need to be replaced. If you want to treat

yourself, step up from the handle the manufacturer provides and buy yourself something that's easier to grip, but made for that brand of cartridge. Avoid anything with more than three blades if you want precision – for instance, around the sideburns.

There are two main alternatives to the cartridge: the safety razor and the straight razor. 'Safety' seems an odd word to use for a device that requires you to handle super-sharp metal blades. Basically you will buy a razor to fit these, and screw them into place. Safety razors go very close, but they require a steady hand and a man who really knows his face – otherwise, expect to be dabbing yours with a tissue paper. If you can get it right, though, they are elegant, old-fashioned and affordable – working out much cheaper than a cartridge habit. If you want to experiment, start with a butterfly safety razor, which are designed to make it easy to insert new blades.

Safety razors are kid's toys by comparison to the straight razor. This is the horrifying implement you may have seen wielded by a barber, or a homicidal maniac looking to carve you up like a pumpkin. Needless to say, these are best left to the adventurous and the pros.

There's a huge number of creams, gels and foams available. As before, avoid perfumed products where possible. Don't bother with foam from a can – light and fluffy, it does little to comfort your face or soften the hairs. Opt instead for something more emollient, which you can rub on by hand. The act of lathering up helps prepare the hairs for shaving.

The ultimate cream is the one you prepare yourself with a shaving brush of badger hair and a mug of shaving soap. Frothing the soap with the brush produces a rich lather that helps your shave, and the application cuts down the chance of in-growing hairs.

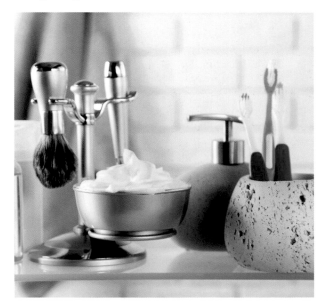

HOW TO
SHAVE

Once your face is prepared – hair softened, cream applied – you are ready. Shave in the direction in which your hair grows – usually, downwards. Some parts of the face may feature hairs growing in several directions at once. Run your hand over your face before you start and feel where the hairs are pointing.

Over time you will learn an order and direction that works for you – start with trying to go with (not against) the grain as much as possible. Against-the-grain shaving has its fans, since it gets you closer – but skin may be more irritated/ nicked, so it is not for the sensitive. Cover your face in soap/foam and leave for 1–2 minutes to soften.

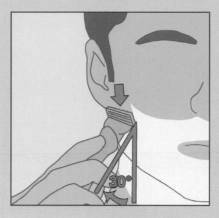

1 | Hold the razor at an angle of 30 degrees. There is no right order, but it may help to begin at the sideburns, starting from the top and moving down to the jaw line.

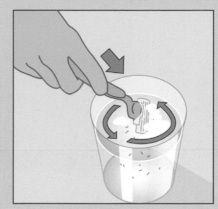

2 | As you shave, rinse the razor regularly – under the tap or in a glass of warm water. After the sideburns are done, move to the moustache.

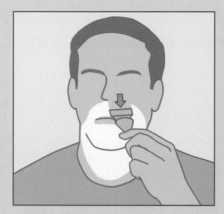

3 | Again going with the direction of growth, shave all the moustache area, usually downwards but sometimes outwards horizontally. Now move to the cheeks, moving from the outside of your face inwards, and again with the direction of growth. You can pull the skin tight in problem areas to help, but don't be tempted to lean on the blade – maintain light pressure throughout.

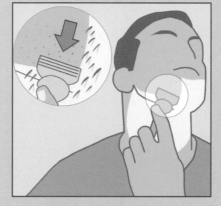

4 | Once the face is finished move on to the chin, chin hairs are often the most tough, so it makes sense to leave these to soften under the cream for the longest. Move downwards over the chin line and down the neck. Right beneath the jawline can be a problem area because it is contoured, if so try pulling the skin on your cheek upwards so the skin that is right beneath the jawline moves up and is easier to access.

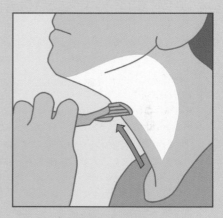

5 | Finish underneath the chin with a mixture of downward and upward strokes. You don't have to get a perfect shave first time – feel free to come back for any difficult bits. Running your hand over your face will help you locate any remaining bristles. Stubborn areas may require you to go against or across the grain. Apply more cream if you need to. Finish with a few cold splashes of water, then pat your face dry with a clean towel. Follow with a moisturiser or shaving balm.

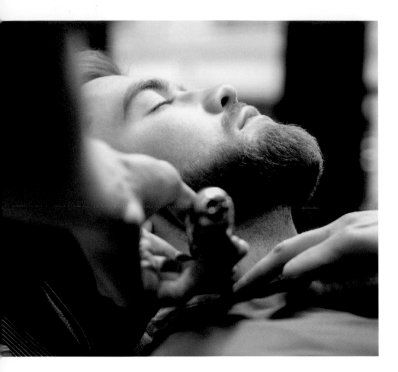

To beard or not to beard

Once upon a time, beards were the province of geography teachers and lumberjacks. At some point that changed, and at the time of writing, stylish young men in city streets proudly model facial hair made fashionable by Arctic scientists and Victorian explorers. It may be that we have hit 'peak beard' – but once men have had a taste of what can be achieved, it's unlikely they will ever go back.

Not growing a beard

Not all men can grow a beard, and not all men should. It's not fair, but there it is. Some men have patchy, wiry, sparse facial hair, bits that don't join up, or unexpectedly ginger chin hair. If this is you, don't despair, just work with what you've got. A full beard may not work, but you may have the potential for sideburns, a goatee or a moustache. If not, accept it, move on and learn to shave properly (see 'How to shave' on p113) – a scraggly beard is a bad look.

Growing a beard

If you are more hirsute, you may want to give the beard thing a go. Before you pack away your razor, however, it's helpful to understand what is required both during and after the growing period.

◆ Start by giving yourself a good cleanse and a shave. You are preparing the ground that will soon be covered by a thick forest, so take care and time and do it right.
◆ It will itch an awful lot at first. Hang tough. The first week is the worst. Washing with a beard shampoo will help, as will exfoliating.

◆ If you are working during this period, you may want to keep your clothing standards extra sharp. Wearing a tie will make it clear you haven't given up, but are trying something new.
◆ Remove stray hairs on cheekbones and keep your neck trimmed – but beware being too neat, or doing too much shaping.
◆ It will take about a month for you to have a real idea of what you've got to work with, and reach something like full beard.
◆ Gaps in a beard or lighter hair can be disguised by using coloured moustache wax – shoe polish for your facial hair, it colours in and fills in, but does need regular application and a light touch – too much and you will look like a kid playing pirates.
◆ It isn't true that shaving will make your beard come back fuller, so don't try this approach.

Maintaining

Think of a beard as an extension of your hair, and deserving of as much attention. Since it also a part of your face, it needs a gentle approach.

Maintain a good-looking beard that is free of crumbs by using a cleaning routine. Comb it out daily and wash it regularly – ideally with a specialist product. Don't forget to look after the skin under the beard. Having a regular exfoliate as part of your facial routine helps slough off any dead skin hiding under the hairs – be sure to rinse properly. Apply a moisturiser for your face – lighter products will be less likely to linger in the hairs. Follow up with a beard oil or balm and comb through.

Keeping your beard tidy will depend on the natural shape of your growth. At the very least, you will want to keep your cheekbones free of any stray hairs that have wandered – this will make the main growth look sharper. A shaved neck provides contrast against a bearded chin, but looks fussy and can give you a visual double chin. A sensible middle-ground option is to buy a beard clipper and trim it lightly, fading from around the Adam's apple down.

If you bought a beard trimmer and have a steady hand you can keep your beard to a length that works for you. Alternatively, find a barber who is good with beards and book yourself a regular trim. Moustaches should be combed down and trimmed (scissors are good for this job) across the top of the lip.

Oh, and check yourself after every meal. Not all your friends or dates will tell you there is salmon in your beard.

Five o'clock shadow

The hint of a beard is a good compromise for the man who doesn't want to go full facial – and is often cited as the most attractive look a man can sport. Worn with appropriately

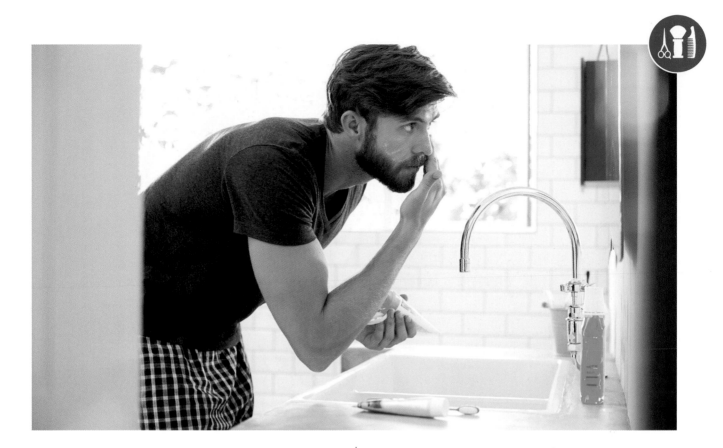

smart contrasting clothes, it is more rugged than scruffy, as suitable for an office as a fishing trip. It's a good choice for men who want to take the edge off a clean-cut look – provided they have the coverage. If your facial hair sprouts sparsely, it may not work.

Follow the aforementioned styling tips. Since the contrast between shaved and hairy is less pronounced than with a full beard, you can afford to clean up the neck a bit – but beware the over-sculpted look. The object is to appear rugged, not like you took a ruler to it. Use a beard trimmer to keep the hairs at an even length and to fade the neck growth.

Tidy brows and nostrils

Your aim in approaching eyebrow care is to hit the middle ground between the monobrow and the teeny tiny precision brows – to tidy it up, but leave it looking natural.

It's easier to trim eyebrows after a hot shower. Exfoliate the area, then comb the hairs upwards. For a simple trim, use a sharp, small pair of scissors to cut off the hairs that protrude above the natural shape of your brow.

For the removal of strays, or for thinning, use a good pair of tweezers (never a razor, or a wax – it'll make them look drawn-on) and a mirror – ideally, a magnifying mirror so you can see what you are doing. Pinch a hair near the base and give a short, sharp yank. If in doubt, remove fewer hairs – you will be surprised how quickly you can clear the thicket.

Totally reshaping your brows is best left to a professional. If you're ignoring this advice and doing this at home, think

of it instead as a tidy-up, and steer clear of trying to create a defined shape, such as an arch. Don't aim to make the brows match perfectly. Thin out the hairs in the middle of a monobrow, rather than removing them entirely.

While you've got the special mirror and sharp scissors out, sort your nasal fur too. Nose hairs should always be kept short, so they don't extend beyond the confines of your nose. Never pluck them (risk of infection) – instead use a trimmer, or scissors (with care).

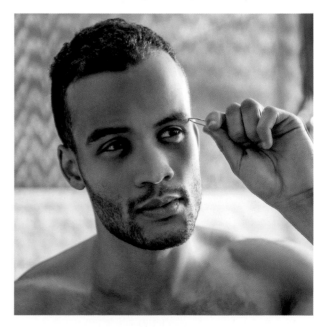

Manage body hair

Again, the balance when trimming body hair lies midway between doing too much and too little. Once you start removing body hair, you may not stop – and smooth-chested Ken doll is not a good look for a real human, unless you are a sportsman and it is beneficial/required.

◆ Chest: The sensible middle ground is a trim with a good pair of clippers. Go in the direction of the hair growth, moisturise afterwards, and go easy at first. Think about the contrast between face and body – if you've got a bit of beard, keep some hair.
◆ Back/shoulders: Hair on these areas is not a good look, by general agreement, although some women claim to like it. You can't do this yourself. Book a wax.
◆ Downstairs: Less is more. You don't want to look like the aforementioned Ken doll, but neither do you want bush creeping out of your undies. A quick go with the clippers to thin out is a good compromise.
◆ Penis/balls: Really? OK. Some men do defoliate here, believing it is aesthetically pleasing/makes their junk look bigger. But since that means passing a sharp object over your most prized possessions – and a lot of itchy sensations afterwards – think carefully.
◆ Bum: If sir insists. A steady hand and a trimmer are required, or get it done at the same time as the back.

Foot care

If you want to truly horrify a prospective partner, ignore your feet. Let them do their thing. Grow big, nasty toenails that rip the duvet and punch holes in your delicate socks. Let the smell ripen and mature. Or don't. Stop taking your feet for granted. Show them some love. Wash them thoroughly, and if you have fragrance issues, give them an occasional soak. Dry them properly, and if you are a talcum man, give them a little powder. Trim the toenails carefully – best after

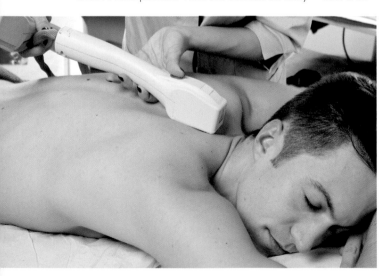

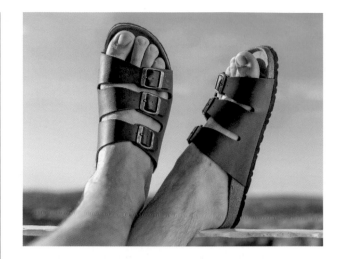

a bath or shower – and ensure that you cut them straight across. Keep a foot file, and make it a weekly habit to sand off any dry skin. Applying a little lotion will keep them soft and supple. Once in a while, take them on a trip to a professional. A podiatrist will treat your feet, gently, and with better tools and more experience than you have.

How to give yourself a manicure

A man can dress well, fix his hair right, smell good – but if he has long, cracked and/or dirty fingernails, it's game over. Learn to look after your hands and nails.

1 First clip, leaving a strip of white at the end of the nail. Don't go too close to the quick, or cut off the corners.
2 File gently with an emery board, in one direction, smoothing off the nail and gently rounding the corners.
3 Snip off any loose peels of skin around the nail with a sharp pair of scissors or a 'cuticle nipper' and gently shape any scruffy cuticles by pushing any skin back, preferably with a special little wooden cuticle stick.
4 Wash, rinse and moisturise.

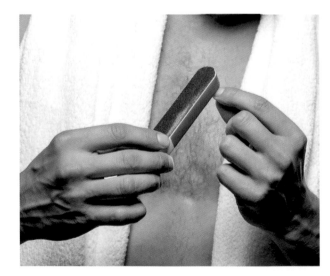

SMELLING OF ROSES

How a man smells can have a profound influence on the impact he makes on the world. It is invisible, subtle and works on a subconscious level. A powerful weapon – used in the wrong way, it can have disastrous results.

Deodorant

Every man needs a deodorant, but not all men need an anti-perspirant. The first gets rid of the smell from your armpits, the second stops up the pores so the sweat can't get through in the first place. Whichever you choose, it's a good idea to go for a non-perfumed product. A man's fragrance should reflect him and the care he has put into choosing something that announces him to the world. You do not want that fragrance competing with whatever stuff they put in a deodorant to justify calling it 'Jungle Heat' or similar. If you have problems, such as regularly sweat-drenched armpits – consider a specialist product. It's strong stuff, so don't overdo it.

Find your fragrance

It may take you time to find a fragrance you love. Buy samples, try things on in the shop (be sure you aren't wearing any fragrance for this), ask people's views. In the shop, spray a little on the small cards until you find something you like enough to try on your skin. What works on paper may work differently when it connects with you. Don't buy straight away – give it an hour or so to develop on your skin. Make a note of what you like, research what else has that quality or ingredient, and if you have the money, begin a small collection. Start with some classics – the contrast between a young man and an old-school fragrance can be a real winner.

Wearing fragrance

Fragrance should always be applied lightly – the worst thing a man can do is to drown himself in perfume. Dab a little at the neck and wrists, where increased blood flow near the skin means constant low heat. For a longer-lasting effect, spritz a small amount on the centre of your chest. Start small – better to underdo than overdo. Do not spritz more than three times, max.

Fragrance products, in order of strength:
◆ Eau de Parfum: The strong stuff.
◆ Eau du Toilette: Toilet water. A little more diluted. More staying power than EDC, below.
◆ Eau du Cologne: More diluted still, and therefore subtle.
◆ Aftershave: Weakest whiff of the lot. Mostly for splashing on, rather than smelling nice.

Five classic fragrances

Obviously there are thousands of perfumes out there, and you must find the one(s) that work for you, but here are a few (in no particular order) that have stood the test of time and have widespread appeal:

Green Irish Tweed, Creed
Woody, green, this is a powerful, expensive, manly yet sophisticated smell.

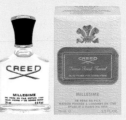

Eau Sauvage, Christian Dior
The 1966 fragrance that notoriously knocked les femmes for six. Very elegant, very sexy, very French. Lemon, basil, rosemary, vetiver.

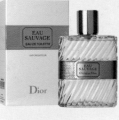

Blenheim Bouquet, Penhaligon's
The classic, subtle, discreet, austere British scent. Citrus and pine. As worn by Winston Churchill.

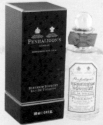

Acqua di Parma
Old-school Mediterranean. Very Italian. Citrus, rosemary, lavender. A summer smell.

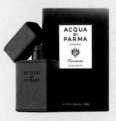

Old Spice
OS has made a comeback as the best of the old-school cheap fragrances. It has lasted because it works. Very manly – spices such as nutmeg and star anise, orange and lemon, with florals and cinnamon/vanilla.

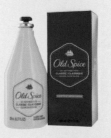

PROFESSIONAL HELP

This chapter has detailed the many measures a man can take to look after his body, mind and facial hair. There is, however, a limit to what a guy can achieve on his own, and some jobs are best left to those who specialise in them – the professionals. It's not enough to just plonk your money down; to get the very best work you have to be very clear what you want – or you will have zero chance of getting it.

Hairdresser/barber

Neither the barber nor the hairdresser is any 'better' than the other, necessarily. The cut of a good barber will be as reliably excellent as that of a good hairdresser, but their focus will be different. A barber will mostly cut men's hair. He will be adept with the razor and the clipper, may offer a shaving service, and should know how to offer straightforward, old-school styles without fuss. It's likely he will work at a decent pace, and won't expect to be spending an hour on your style.

A hairdresser will reach for the scissors before the clippers, and will spend time talking to you about your needs, and delivering them. They generally won't specialise in men's hair, and unless you've gone for a cheap high street chain, they will not begrudge talking to you about what you want, and offering advice on how to achieve it.

Which you choose depends on you and your hair. Start by working out what kind of cut you want.

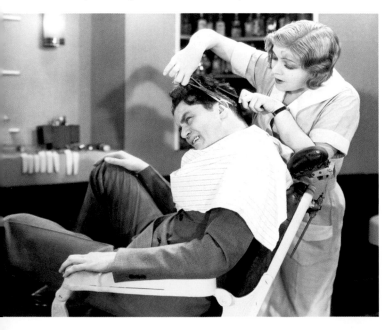

Choosing a hair style

If you are aiming for a straightforward, tidy, old-school look – a crop, a crew cut, a quiff, a short-back-and-sides – then the authentic barber will do the job right. A hairdresser can deliver those cuts, but it is a bit like walking into a cocktail bar and ordering a pint.

There is lots of advice available for men who aren't sure what hairstyle to go for. However, there are so many variables at play – height, hair type, face shape, etc – that a one-size-fits-all approach doesn't make much sense.

Start by narrowing it down to what can be achieved with what you've got. There is no point dreaming of a slick, sculpted quiff if you have tight curls, and thick wavy hair will always want to do its own thing. Hair can be treated with heat and chemicals, cut and shaped and bent to your will – but the more work it is, the more likely it is that it will look forced. A hairdresser will tell you that everyone always wants someone else's hair – accepting what you've got is the first step towards making it look good. Think about upkeep too – if you aren't the kind of guy who likes to spend time primping, get something that's low maintenance. A French crop (short, textured, brushed forwards) suits most men and can be styled in 30 seconds.

Get advice. Ask a hairdresser/barber what look might suit you. They can tell you what the non-starters are, and what will work for your face – see opposite. Keep an eye out for haircuts that appeal to you, in magazines, TV, movies. Who looks slick? Take a picture into the salon/shop, and ask them whether they can deliver it (much easier than learning the appropriate hairdressing terms).

Whatever you do, don't end up having the same hairstyle, time after time, because you are wary of risking it. A new style is the quickest, cheapest way to revolutionise your look, and if you take a chance, the odds are it will pay off. And if it doesn't, just get it cropped short, or grow it back out again. Because there is nothing that says more about a man's lack of imagination than the words 'just a trim'.

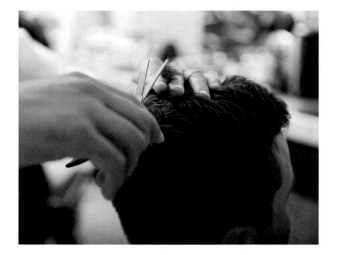

Face types

You can spend hours measuring your face, but honestly you can get a good idea just by looking at it – or even better, asking your barber/hairdresser. They've seen a lot of heads. Part of the job of an effective hairstyle is to soften or help define your natural looks.

◆ Men with oval or round faces should avoid haircuts that make them appear more spherical. Ovals might opt instead for something angular – shorter sides and a sharp side parting with a bit of length on top both work. For the rounder-faced fellow, the higher hair of a squared-off quiff will help to elongate. Fringes may add unwelcome width, but you might try keeping the sides short and contrasting with an angular fringe swept from the side. A well-shaped beard can add a bit of strength to a soft jawline.

◆ Square-faced men have the reverse issue – instead of looking for sharp lines to break up the smooth edges, they may want to import some softness by going longer all over. Conversely, if you can carry it, a very short, tight cut will accentuate strong chiselled features, though depending on your face it can look a little extreme. Squares are considered the masculine shape with the licence to get away with more, so feel free to experiment. If your jawline is just too macho for words, you can soften it with a light beard.

◆ Rectangles are longer, and you will want to hide that length – so avoid the short sides recommended for the round/square-faced chaps. Look to add width with a bit of length and volume across the piece, with a fringe that falls across the face. Softer styles take away from the block-shaped head look.

◆ Triangular faces appear wider at the bottom than the top – compensate with some extra volume, and keep it full and thick at the sides to sculpt the head shape.

◆ Diamond-shaped faces will benefit from some length on top, and a soft fringe may balance out the angularity.

Tattooist

If there is a life decision to take your time over, it is this one. Think about who you were five years ago. Remember that guy? The ridiculous stuff he was into? The girl he was going to love forever? That's how future you is going to be feeling about the guy you are now. You should also be aware that tattoos can evoke a certain reaction in some people, and at some point this could work against you.

If you are set on ink and of age, you have two big decisions: who and what. If you are going old-school tattoo, you might consider a classic – but let it be your choice, customised to you and what you like. NB Tattoos featuring names and faces are rarely a good idea, given what life throws at you and how people can and do change.

When you have an idea of what you want, it'll help you find the person to do it. Look for the specialist, the artist, the one whose work really speaks to you. Social media is a boon, as are personal recommendations. Be prepared to travel, and to pay. Cheap is not a good idea. When you've got a shortlist, check out the artist and their work, in more detail and in person. Check too the hygiene standards of the parlour (and it has to be a proper shop, none of this backroom bullshit) because Hepatitis is as much a risk as a crooked tat. Make sure you see the used needles being disposed of, and new ones opened.

When you've found the artist, talk through the idea and see what you can come up with together. Then wait. Pin a print of the art somewhere you will always see it – on the wall by the bed – and live with it. No rush. Is it getting on your nerves yet? If the answer is no, and your best guess is that it will stay that way, then book yourself in.

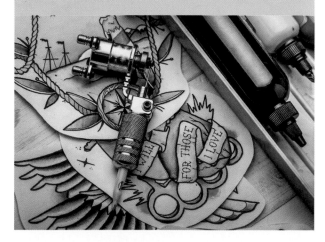

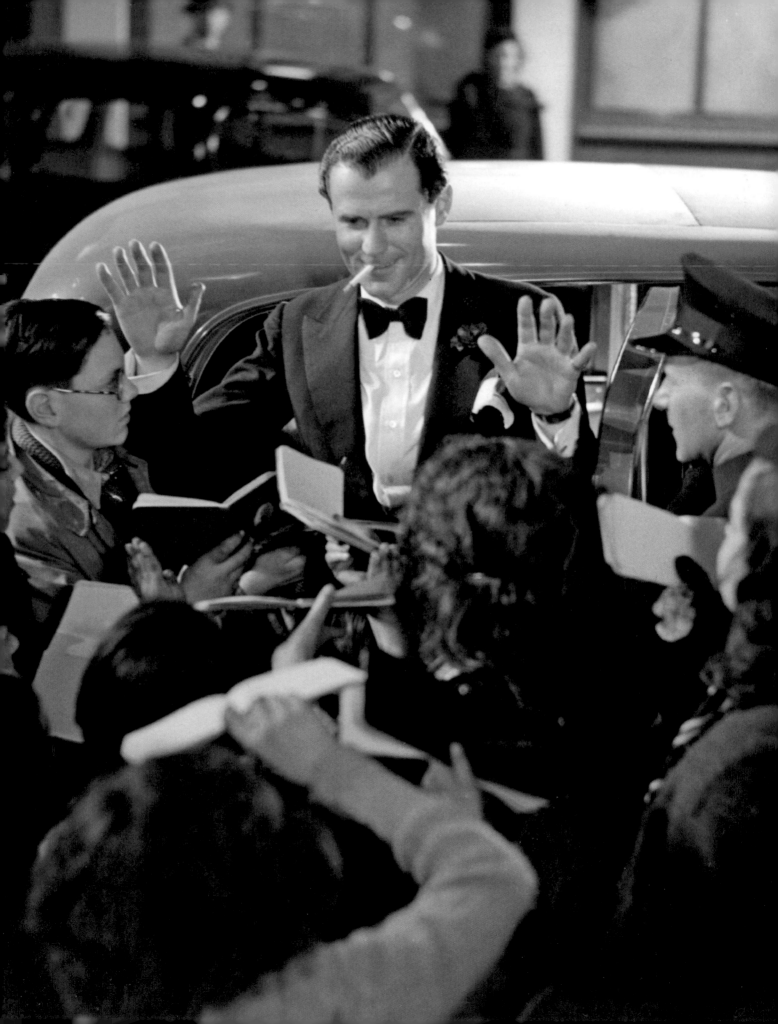

CHAPTER 5

SOCIAL SUCCESS

Of all the talents a man can master, none is more vital to a happy, full existence than his social skills. The world, as you may have noticed, has other people in it. How you navigate your way around them will define your life and how others see you. Learning how to talk to anyone, about anything (and to really listen to their replies) will make you and your time on earth much more interesting.

HOW TO TALK TO ANYONE

Learning to talk to people is a vital life skill, invaluable in almost any situation you might find yourself in: work, love, travel, a lift. Like all skills, some may have a natural affinity for this, making it look easy, but that doesn't mean it can't be learned, or that everyone who has it was born that way.

Anyone who claims they've walked into a room full of strangers without feeling at least a mild sense of panic is either lying or horribly over-confident. For the rest of us, it's a daunting prospect.

The quickest way to get over fear is to confront it, directly, so if you find the idea of starting a conversation with a random stranger difficult, do it anyway, as often as possible. And take heart from the fact that (like many skills) confident communication can be faked until it becomes second nature. With a few simple tricks anyone can learn to manage their nerves and find meaningful conversation and useful networking.

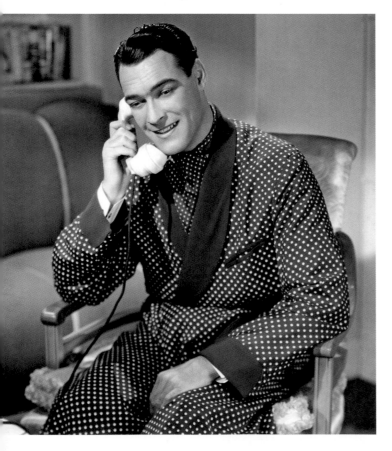

Listening

The first rule of talking is: don't. Listen. Your aim in most social and professional situations involving strangers is not to dazzle them with your hilarious anecdotes, but to leave a positive impression of an interesting person they enjoyed spending time with. The quickest path to that goal is by asking questions and listening to the answers.

Adjusting your attitude helps. Look at a sea of strangers as an opportunity. True fact: strangers are interesting, and you will learn something more about people and the world with every exchange. So, next time you take a taxi, make it your mission to find out where the driver is from and what the food is like there. You will discover something. Even if it's only not to eat lunch in Scunthorpe.

Party/work do

In a party or work social environment where there are a lot of people you don't know, don't look for a familiar face, or a repeat of an interaction you have already had. Instead, scan the room for someone on their own. Odds are they will welcome a conversation. Any kind of opening will do, including 'hello'. It's like diving off a high board – thinking about doing it is way harder than actually doing it. Step off the edge and say something. If you can't think of anything, start with what you have in common: how do they know the host, isn't it hot, how's the food?

Make eye contact. Smile. Do what you can to relax – breathe, stay still. Ask open-ended questions. You don't want to sound like an interrogator, but you do want to seem (and be) genuinely interested in who they are, where they are from, what they do for a living. Follow up with questions about how they got into the line of work, or what they like about it. Get them to explain it to you – everyone loves being a teacher/guide. At some point in the interaction, introduce yourself with a smile, a handshake, and eye contact. Make an effort to remember

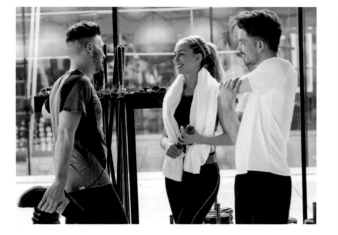

their name – repeating it back to them helps mark you out as someone who is interested, who pays attention.

There's nothing wrong with a bit of mild disagreement but in most social contexts you will want to avoid the kind of full-blown row that can arise when strangers discuss politics. And remember where you are – if it is a work do, hold off on frank stories about that time you were in Tijuana.

At some point, even if you haven't had a disagreement, you'll want to move on to someone new, which can prove tricky if you find yourself stuck with one person and no 'out'. You don't need an elaborate excuse, just an 'excuse me' and a 'very nice to meet you (insert name here)'. Then make a beeline for a new stranger – again, ideally someone solo. Carrying a second drink enables you to make an exit in the direction of whichever imaginary person it is supposedly for.

Chatting up

Chatting someone up uses the same skills and techniques described above, but may get more personal more quickly, depending on your confidence levels and the mutual chemistry. As with all confidence issues, the trick is to act

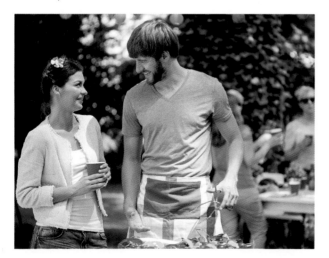

Meeting the parents

Meeting your partner's parents for the first time is an unnerving experience. It's easy to feel the pressure, as if you are being assessed from head to toe, weighed up for your prospects and judged on whether you are worthy of their precious offspring. That's because you are.

Do what you can to let go of the nerves at this point and don't try too hard to impress. Just be sincere, polite and warm. Do some research on the family beforehand so you know the basics – jobs, siblings, interests, etc. Dress with care and carry a peace offering if you can – flowers are a nice touch. Be prepared to give an account of yourself (eg your background and career/life plans). Don't expect rejection, but be aware that parents can be protective, and judgemental – don't take it personally.

Keep the conversation light and away from flashpoints – you don't want a run-in over politics. If it does get argumentative, keep a cool head and let your partner sort it out (if they choose not to stand up for you, there may be an issue). You're likely to be seeing these people for several years to come – so make an effort to get along, no matter what.

like you feel cool until you find you do. There is a fine line between mutually enjoyable flirtation and harassment. Not all men are capable of seeing the distinction. Don't be that guy. If someone isn't into talking to you, let it go and move on. See p154 for more on romantic communications.

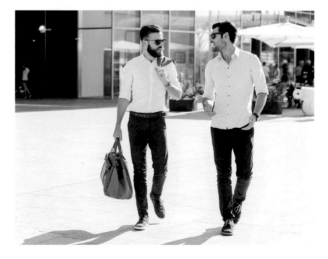

WORKPLACE SKILLS

Whatever your job, whatever your plans for your future career, you can't thrive without putting in some considered effort. Learning how to effectively communicate with colleagues, to send emails that represent you properly, to speak in public and deal with drama will pay off in the long run. Even if your current situation is temporary, doing some preparation, watching your back and being prepared to work your ass off is a good strategy.

Interviews

It doesn't matter how experienced you are, how perfect you are for the role – if you can't perform in an interview, you won't get the opportunity to show it. Interviewing is a skill, and it can be learned.

◆ Don't expect to just rock up and get the position. Even if you have a good idea that you are the man for the job, take it as a challenge and rise to the occasion.

◆ Research, research, research. Learn everything you can about the job and the company. Google like a maniac. What are the company's values? What challenges do they face? You are looking to demonstrate knowledge about the business. If you can talk to the current post-holder, do.

◆ More research. Don't stop there. Who is doing the interview? What's their background? Who else could tell you something you don't know about the gig?

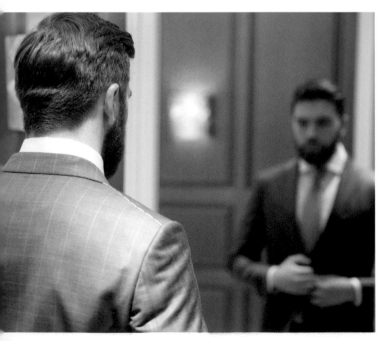

◆ Practise. In most interview situations you will need to deliver to a checklist of the skills, experience and aptitudes of the person they want – as spelled out in the job description. You need stories demonstrating you tick all those boxes and more – examples of how you have used your skills to make things better. Make them short and punchy – what was the problem, how did you fix it, what was the resolution? Try them aloud.

◆ If you are in the early stages of your career, stress your enthusiasm and motivation, and think creatively about answers to questions about experience. It doesn't have to be restricted to work.

◆ Get there early. Plan the journey, make sure you have what you need. Don't go in hungry, thirsty or so caffeinated you can't speak.

◆ Dress well. If you want to be taken seriously, dress seriously, in a style that echoes the standards of the workplace.

◆ Relax. Try breathing exercises, or picturing the interviewers in their underwear – whatever allows you to be yourself and project confidence.

◆ Smile. Make eye contact. Keep your body language open, and sit up straight. Listen attentively to what you are being asked. Leaning slightly forwards helps, as does making notes. You can use these if you draw a blank. Bring in a CV if it helps you to refer to it.

◆ When you get the chance to ask questions, drop a good one that shows you know the business, but also demonstrate that you're seeing this as a two way process, you need to find out if this is the right job for you. Don't ask anything that makes you seem like a lightweight. This is not the moment to discuss money – that comes when you get offered the role.

◆ After the interview send an email thanking the interviewer for their time. If you don't get the job, try to find out why. It may be something beyond your control but there is almost always something to learn.

Interview fails

◆ Lateness. Unless there was some major crisis on the train or similar, you aren't coming back from this.
◆ Over excited waffling. Know your stories, get to the point, then shut up.
◆ Bitching. Never ever talk negatively about previous employers, it makes them wonder what you are going to say about them one day.
◆ Ignorance. If you show you know nothing about their business, you are straight on to the no pile.
◆ Lying, or even exaggerating. There's a chance you might get low level bullshit past them, but why take the risk? Stick to what's true and then later you won't have to remember you claimed your interests included sky diving.

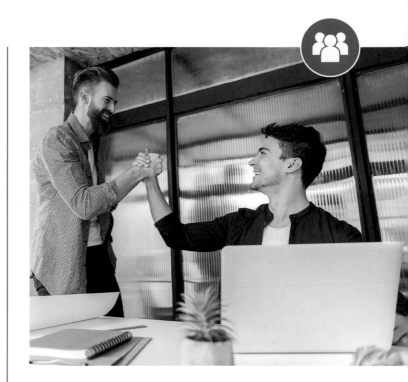

Gaining experience

A majority of employers say young people are not ready for the workplace – even graduates. At any age, a focus on acquiring and honing the basic skills of communication and teamwork can put you ahead. In your early career, nothing beats experience – the wider and more challenging, the better. Whatever you think you might be interested in doing, pursue it – interests can turn into careers, and skills can be developed in all kinds of contexts. Being the guy who referees youth games demonstrates management, diplomacy and judgement under pressure – the kind of details interviewers remember.

Handling a new job

Arriving at a new job can be a daunting experience – many employers will chuck new staff in at the deep end, without giving them much information on what is expected of them. You may find yourself wondering what the hell you are doing. Everyone goes through this. Try to project a sense of confidence – and do what you can to help yourself to feel relaxed. 'Fake it 'til you make it' can be a good strategy, but don't pretend to know more than you do. You'll have a lot to learn – keep your ears and eyes open, ask questions, take notes. If you don't know what you're supposed to be doing, don't be afraid to ask.

◆ Don't feel you always have to take a back seat because you're new – if you see a chance to contribute, seize it.
◆ Manage your expectations – if you are in your early career, you may have to suck it up and do more boring legwork than you'd imagined. The quickest way up is to work hard, even if it isn't what you thought it would be.
◆ Look for ways to help your colleagues. Challenge assumptions by going out of your way for others and challenge yourself by taking on extra duties.
◆ Smile, stay positive and know that it's going to take drive and resilience to get where you want to be.

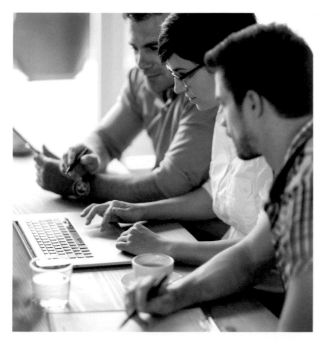

'Try not to become a man of success, but rather try to become a man of value'
Albert Einstein

Managing colleagues

Every workplace has its share of personalities – and unless you are lucky, that will include some difficult types. You have no choice but to deal with these people every day, so avoid conflict wherever possible. The company of overwhelmingly negative people, time-wasters and malicious gossips can bring you down, so if you take the job seriously, keep some distance. Aim to build positive networks instead – take the opportunity to get lunch or coffee with colleagues whose company you enjoy, and learn from them. Bullying is never acceptable – find out what the company policy is and don't be afraid to act on inappropriate behaviour.

Workplace etiquette

◆ Dress like you mean it.
◆ Be on time, and meet your deadlines.
◆ Always stand up when you are introduced to someone and say your full name – expect to shake hands, and remember their name.
◆ Keep your personal life – and personal calls and emails – out of the workplace.
◆ Be polite and aware of others – watch your volume and your language.
◆ Work hard, but watch for burnout – a job is not worth killing yourself for.
◆ Making your boss look good is generally a good strategy.
◆ If you are genuinely sick, don't come in. Especially if you may be contagious – your colleagues will not thank you. (NB a hangover doesn't count).
◆ No mobile browsing/taking calls during meetings. Don't mistake looking important with appearing rude, even if senior people make a habit of it.

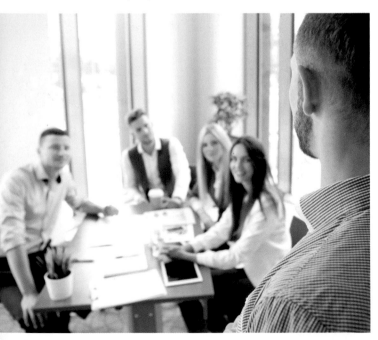

◆ In work-related meal/drink situations, the person who did the inviting is the host and should expect to pay.
◆ If you are at a business meal, don't over-order or guzzle wine – watch what the others do and act accordingly.
◆ Social media can kill your career. Post nothing you wouldn't want your mum to read, and never, ever, bitch about work online.

Giving presentations/public speaking

If there is one test of your nerve and your communications skills it is the presentation/speech – an inevitable rite of passage in many workplace environments. Depending on what you do for a living, you may be able to dodge this for a while, but odds are that at some point, you will be asked to stand in front of a room of strangers and talk, with or without the aid of pictures and charts. If it isn't a formal speech it may just be a crowded meeting and a direct question, or a leaving do for a co-worker. Either way, 20 pairs of eyes focused on you, in silence, has a way of ratcheting up the pressure.

◆ Practise. It's true that some people are good at this, and others find it harder. However, the fundamental difference between a good presentation and otherwise is practise. Deliver it in front of the cat, the mirror, a camera, a friend. Know what you are going to say.
◆ Think about the audience. Tailor what you are delivering to them. What do they want/need to know? What would be useful to them? How long has it been since lunch? Get the message straight. Boil what you are saying down to its purest form. If you could get them to take away one thing from this, what would it be?
◆ Start with a bang. Most crowds need a bit of pepping up – if you have the confidence beginning with a bit of drama makes sure they are listening.
◆ Smile. Breathe. Move around a bit. Make eye contact.
◆ Relax. Adrenaline can cause physical reactions – sweaty palms, nausea, rapid pulse. Slow down, or just stop. You'd be amazed how long a pause you can get away with. Use the time to breathe, deeply and slowly. When you make your point, it will be heard.
◆ Keep a glass of water nearby. It'll help with a dry throat and give you a prop if you need to take a second.
◆ Use notes, but don't just read from the paper.
◆ You're only one person in the room – fixating on your performance takes away your ability to help the others glean the information they need to know. It is guaranteed you've noticed your mistakes more than they have.
◆ Avoid long, boring charts and long, boring speeches. Data is dull. Keep it snappy, varied and interactive. Ask questions, or for a show of hands.
◆ Have a punchy ending. Come up with a line that tells them what you've just told them, and tell them.

EMAIL ETIQUETTE

In the workplace you are judged both on what you say and how you say it – and in many modern workplaces that is more likely to be via email than in person. Make sure your approach to electronic communications represents you properly. Take the care and time you need over emails (and IMs) to ensure they deliver the right message before hitting send.

◆ Get to the point: Know what you want to say and say it, clearly and succinctly. What do you want from the recipient? Don't make them scroll through paragraphs when all they need is a 'yes'.

◆ Assume you are being monitored: Don't email or IM anything to anyone you wouldn't want to see under a picture of you on the front page of the newspapers tomorrow. In emails that means no over-sharing, no confidential information, no dodgy jokes or hilarious memes. Sharing Internet humour makes you look like you have too much time and not enough work.

◆ Keep it civil: Emails lack the softening effect of body language – they can be easily misunderstood, and tempers flare. If someone gets aggressive or impatient with you via electronic comms, sort it out calmly (ideally in person) rather than descending to their level and engaging in a public flame war – no one wins those.

◆ IRL: If you can talk to someone in person or over the phone, do it. If you have to gossip, complain or bitch about your boss or colleagues, do it over coffee.

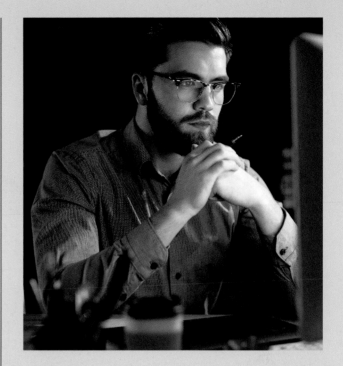

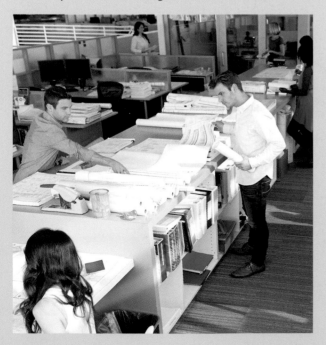

◆ Check spelling and grammar: Check, check and check again. If you aren't familiar with a word, don't use it. Avoid abbreviations and jargon. Read the email you are responding to carefully before replying, and don't ask questions that have been answered.

◆ Don't 'Reply All': Think carefully about distribution. Who needs to see this, and who doesn't? Don't copy senior people in for the sake of it, or to put pressure on the recipient. Equally, don't exclude people who should have a say because you want to cut them out of the conversation. 'BCC' is for people who may not want their email addresses shared widely, not for sneaky grassing or other game playing.

◆ Formality: If in doubt, the formal approach is safer than the informal. Using first names is common practice in most businesses, but tread carefully – if you are addressing the CEO, or a new customer, then 'Dear Ms X' may be better than 'Hi Charlotte'. Unless you know better, play it safe on sign-offs – 'Sincerely' is the height of formality, but if that feels stiff, 'Best regards', 'Best wishes' and 'Thank you' all work.

◆ Don't ignore it: In every industry there are people who never respond to emails, driving everyone else up the wall. It doesn't have to be an instant response – and sometimes a pause to digest and reflect may be more appropriate than a reply in haste. Equally, don't go crazy chasing an immediate response to your email – what is your priority may not be someone else's.

RELATIONSHIP MAINTENANCE

Partners, families and friends can give us the support we need to grow, to deal with the challenges life throws our way and give meaning to our successes. They can also be the source of those hard times, dragging us down and making it feel difficult to move forwards. Either way, a man needs to develop skills to maintain healthy relationships, to manage difficult people, look after loved ones and be sure he is looked after in turn.

Partners

Getting together is the easy part. Without care and attention, relationships suffer. Sitting back and waiting for yours to deliver you everything you need – love, support, affection, sex, understanding, a cup of tea – is not going to work. To get the most from any relationship you need to bring honest communication to the table.

◆ Talk. Be open and honest about what's bothering you and what you want – or need – from your partner. A common complaint about men is that they don't say what's on their mind until it's too late to do anything about it.

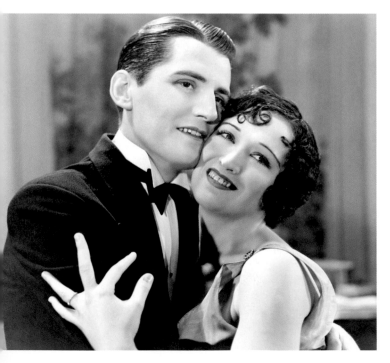

◆ Be realistic. Partners can make life infinitely better. However, no one is going to entirely fix you, or protect you from every lousy thing life throws your way, and all relationships take work.

◆ Acknowledge history. You may be bringing something you experienced with someone else to this relationship. Your new partner can't take responsibility for your past, but they may help you get beyond it.

◆ Practise empathy. It's easy to get caught up in your own feelings. Think about how things feel from the other side.

◆ Accept differences. Don't try to remake someone in your image – let them be themselves, even if they cook pasta the 'wrong' way or like 'bad' TV.

◆ Be yourself. In the early days of a relationship, some people hide the full truth of who they are, thinking it might turn the other person off. Pretending to be someone you are not is an exhausting burden.

◆ Be kind. Recognising a partner has needs that are different from your own also means being aware of the moments when a little thoughtfulness, listening and kindness might help.

◆ Practise listening. People don't tell you their troubles just so that you will give them the answers. Listen to the emotions behind what your partner is saying, and don't feel like you have to give them solutions.

◆ Accentuate the positive. Don't focus on what isn't going well. Notice the good stuff, think about what you enjoy.

◆ Watch your anger levels. You may think you are protecting yourself, but exploding with little notice, making a habit of shouting or sulking can seem aggressive and will leave you isolated. Anger makes it harder to communicate, and get to what's actually bothering you.

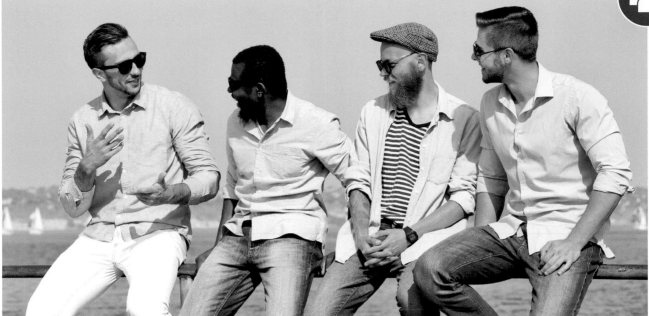

Friends

Friends are the most valuable resource you have – take them for granted and you may find out just how much you rely on them, even if you never discuss anything more meaningful than a golf swing. Take care of them and they will return the favour.

Men are way less likely to talk with friends about their feelings, or emotional developments, such as the fact they just got dumped – announcing that news in the pub may be met with an awkward silence and the offer of another pint. That doesn't mean the company of dudes is any less important in helping us manage. Studies show that men draw support from their friends just as women do, even though we might not be verbalising all the little things. Or, indeed, the big things. Our friends are there for us, though they might not have the words to say it – which is why they offer a pint instead.

Dude night

Men are more likely to let their relationships slide. Make an effort to stay in touch with the guys who have known you from way back when and you will always have a support network. If you haven't seen them for a while, stage a reunion, or get a regular poker night going. Odds are they need it as much as you.

'You never really learn much from hearing yourself speak'
George Clooney

Lady friends

Contrary to what you may have seen in Hollywood movies, men and women can be friends. If you're lucky enough to have a close female friend, you've hit the pal jackpot – their advice will typically give you deeper insight into whatever situation you're in, particularly if it involves a woman. If sex does come up, you'll have to make a difficult call, because it is hard to revert to friendship after knocking boots – but remember it is generally easier to find a lover than a true friend.

Looking after friends

All of the advice here about the kinds of stress, anxiety and darkness a man might experience in life can also apply to his friends. Look after yours, and if it seems like things are going in an unhealthy direction, if you see them becoming isolated, drinking too much or getting aggressive over nothing, act. They may be slow to reach out for help, so if you can sense that something's not right, don't be afraid to ask, rather than wait for the disaster you can see coming. Your role is not therapist or policeman, so hold back from passing judgement, giving them a tough grilling or telling them what to do. Make some time for them, go on a long walk or arrange a camp out so you've got time for sustained conversation. When the right moment comes, explain your concern and listen, ask questions that encourage them to share.

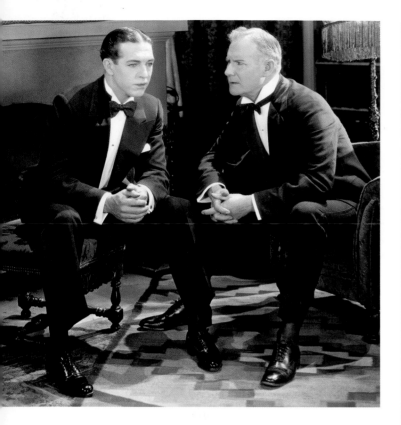

Family

Family circumstances change and relationships develop. Parents that were hugely loving and supportive might get grumpier as they get older, or have health issues that mean they need your support. Siblings that you once fought with can become your best friends, others might follow patterns that have been driving you nuts for decades. Nevertheless, these are the people you have a shared history with and on some level they will always be significant, even if it is just for shared Christmases.

Parents

However old you become, you are still your parents' child. They will look at you and see the baby, toddler and adolescent you once were. You may have to be more patient with them, forgive them for ridiculous behaviour, and make efforts to let them know you still care – call home, make time to visit, arrange events you can do together. The more secure they feel about what is up with you, the less likely they are to attempt to control your adult life. You are

'A man who views the world the same at 50 as he did at 20 has wasted 30 years of his life'
Muhammed Ali

now an adult, dealing with adults, even if that's not how they treat you – they may need to be gently reminded of the fact. Talk to them, openly if you can, about what's going on in your life, your interests. They may be of more help than you expect. If they are driving you away, or up the wall, tell them why.

Siblings

Siblings can offer intense and vital support, or send you insane. If it's the former, enjoy it and make sure you give the same back, if it's the latter pick times to see them outside the family home, do things rather than just meet for a drink. Keep the lines of communication open. You can't change them, but you can change how you deal with them, and opt not to fight fire with fire. Do what you can to encourage positive change, but don't let it make you bitter or crazy if they won't alter their approach or stop being selfish. Set your boundaries, and stick to them. Remember, you might have a tendency to repeat irritating childhood behaviours too.

Children

Fatherhood is, for many guys, the moment they realise they are a man. A grown-up. A responsible adult. There are entire library shelves dedicated to the art of parenting, but it comes down to a simple enough equation. Kids need love, support and shelter. Your job is to provide it.

In a previous generation, being a father meant paying the mortgage and turning up to watch the occasional football game/nativity play. A man could get away with ducking out of bedtimes in favour of the pub. A modern man is more likely to feel pity for those guys than envy – they didn't know what they were missing. Today, a father is expected (rightly) to get involved and pull his weight with every aspect of parenting, work that is as rewarding as it is

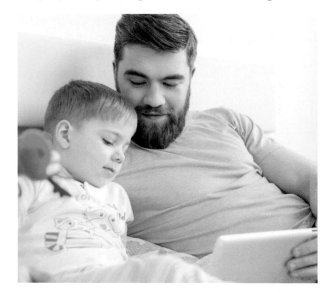

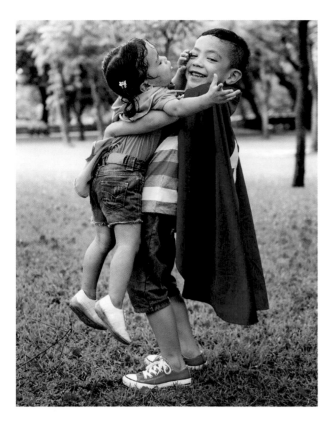

knackering. There are no jobs that are inherently fenced off for mums – other than breast-feeding, but even that can be managed with a breast pump and a bottle.

Being a good dad means delivering on all the things your own father did well, and all the things he didn't. What you want now comes second to what they need – the guy who holds on to self-indulgent habits from his young and free days needs to learn to let go. Most fathers know that there is nothing to beat the feeling that comes with spending time with your kids, because they remember how good it was to spend time with their own dads.

Build them up. Nothing changes a person's life for the better than self-esteem, and that belief starts with parents who encourage and support. Do the practical stuff you need to do to make sure they are safe whatever happens, such as seat belts for them and life insurance for you. Teach them the skills they need to get through life, such as how to deal with people and how to manage money. Work with, not against their mum (even if you aren't together) and show them that a real man respects women. Equality means you don't have to split being good cop/bad cop by gender. Nothing makes a man a feminist quicker than having a daughter – wanting the best opportunities for her may open your eyes to an unequal world.

Enjoy it. We are the generation of guys who get to take part in our kids' childhoods, and even though the work/life balance can be tough, we are damned lucky to be there to see them grow up.

Dealing with feeling

Many men have been taught to suppress emotion, because some people believe that's just what a guy does. He doesn't cry, he doesn't moan, he doesn't say what's wrong but sucks it up. The truth is, men feel emotions no less deeply or truly than women – but they may find it harder to identify those feelings, or deal with them. They may seek other outlets for the raging emotional currents – screaming at the football, an intense approach to work, a religious devotion to pumping weights.

Handling emotion can be particularly difficult if you don't have much experience of expressing feelings, or you've kept it zipped so long it tends to explode out of you without warning – or if you have a partner who would prefer you to man up and clam up. Admitting you've got more on your plate than you can cope with alone is a good start. Everyone needs someone who will listen, and ideally remain patient while you find your way to explaining what's up. If you can't find a friend, family member or colleague for the role, and you're struggling to manage your thoughts and feelings, think about consulting a professional. Counsellors and therapists can help you understand and articulate raging emotions and teach you how to manage and express them.

There's a place for withdrawing, to have a good mull on the situation – a common male habit – but beware how this comes across, and take care not to indulge it at the cost of the relationship.

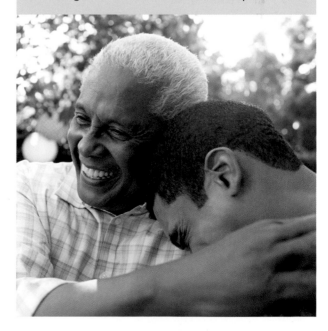

SOCIAL SKILLS

Social skills are life talents for navigating the modern era. Your great-grandfather had to know how to dance the foxtrot and load a rifle, his great-grandfather had to know how to split logs and skin a rabbit. You have to programme a satnav and manage a Twitter account. The skills have changed as the role of man and the expectations placed on him has shifted, but they remain essential to your success.

Buying gifts

A well-chosen present tells someone that you care and know them well enough to have some insight into what would make them really happy. Start noting ideas in advance, look for clues on the things they covet, but would never treat themselves to. Think creatively, about activities and trips as well as products.

Romantic gifts

As a very general rule of thumb when buying a romantic gift, small but luxurious works: high-end accessories from designer shops – lingerie, fragrance, handbags, all of which may be safer than clothes because then you don't have to negotiate fit; expensive chocolates; jewellery. If you're thinking clothes, check their closet for the right size, and keep the receipt – enclose it with the gift, in an envelope.

Think of something that reflects your time together or a shared interest. If it is an anniversary or birthday, do not go practical. On paper she may need a lawnmower, in practice she will not be happy to unwrap one.

NB Not everyone likes surprises, particularly those that cause upheaval – eg the weekend in Paris he won't have been able to pack for, the spa evening after she's just been to the hairdresser's. Approach with care, and don't assume the big romantic gesture will go down exactly as planned.

Choosing flowers

A man will always get credit for buying flowers – but don't expect to see anyone's face light up at the sight of a few wilted blooms from the supermarket. The best way to get good flowers is to find a florist. Look for somewhere with a bit of elegance and ask their advice. Tell them who it is for, the occasion and what your budget is. They are creative people, who like a challenge. Think about the recipient's taste – are they elegant, modern, old-fashioned, do they have a favourite colour? Think too about where they will go – what's the decor like? If money is really tight, find the cheapest flowers in the shop, buy five stems, and have the florist wrap them with greenery.

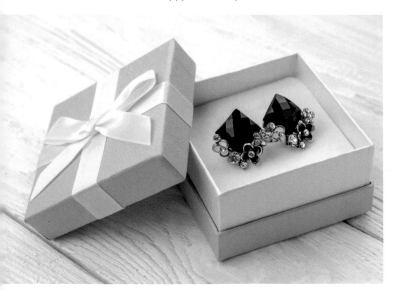

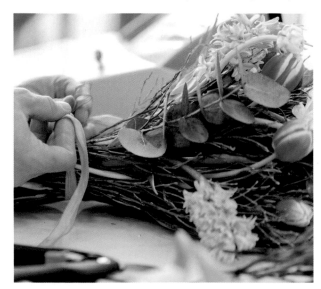

HOW TO
WRAP A PRESENT

You may be able to get a gift wrapped by the shop – but doing it yourself will win points. These instructions show how to wrap a rectangular-shaped gift, for a square-shaped gift use a square piece of paper. Before you begin, cut yourself a few small lengths of tape and leave them where you can reach them.

Equipment
Adhesive tape, scissors, paper, ruler, ribbon, patience.

◆ To curl the ends of ribbon place it in between your thumb and one side of a pair of scissors, then gently pull the ribbon through until you reach the end.
◆ If your folded flap of paper is so long it is dangling over the end, fold it in to square it off, or cut it so it lines up nicely with the end of the side of the gift.

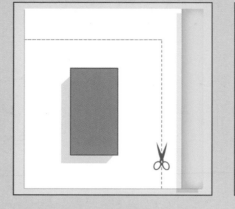

1 Roll out the paper across a clean table top and set the box flat on it. Pull the paper all the way round the box to ensure it is long enough to cover the whole package – give yourself at least a couple of inches' excess. Mark the amount you need, then cut, using the ruler for a straight line. If you don't have a ruler, a straight fold will help guide the scissors. Hold the paper taut while you cut.

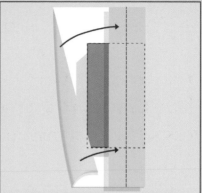

2 Place the box in the centre of the paper, one of the short sides towards you. Pull first one long side of paper over to cover half of the box, then the other side, so that they overlap neatly. Secure with a piece of tape. You now have a burrito shape.

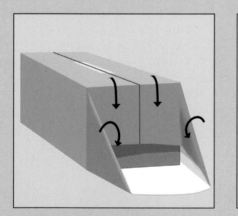

3 Now you need to tidy away the ends of paper protruding over the shorter sides of the box. You're aiming for an envelope effect. Start at one end (making sure you don't push the present and make the sides uneven) and press the paper on one side towards the middle of the uncovered section.

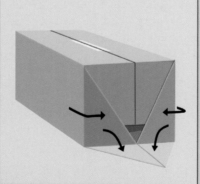

4 Make a fold in the overhanging bit of paper, and the bit underneath, so that the crease will angle in like an envelope, fold up and stick down with tape. Repeat for the other end.

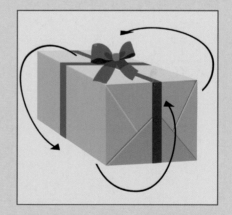

5 Pass the ribbon around the box, cross the ends underneath and pull both ends back round over the other sides of the box back to the top again. Tie a neat bow. If you are not really into pretty bows and glittery finishes customize the gift accordingly. Try brown paper, string and a sprig of greenery for a more natural, but no less impressive look.

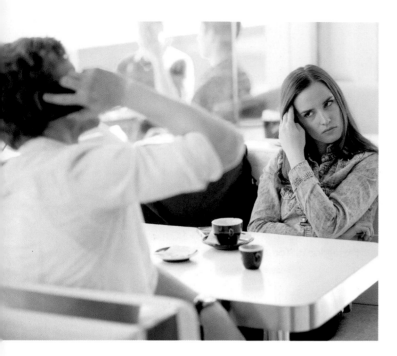

Thrive on social media

Social media is an undeniable fact of our era, but you don't have to let your use of it define you. If the first thing you do in the morning is check your phone, it might be time to give yourself a digital detox and focus on the real world.

The ease of social media brings great risk – it is now possible to utterly screw your reputation and career armed only with a phone, 2 minutes and a lack of foresight. Rule number one is to set your standards high. Not everything you think about posting, or tweeting, has to be posted or tweeted. Daisy Buchanan, author of *How to Be A Grown Up*, offers words so wise they should be tattooed on every man's tweeting thumb: 'Do not tweet ragefully, drunkenly, or spitefully – and do not say anything you would be ashamed to repeat in front of Michelle Obama/the Queen.'

Social media guidelines

◆ If you are likely to say something that might make you blush tomorrow, put the phone in your pants drawer, do something else, go to bed. See how you feel in the morning. The phone is in your pants drawer, by the way.

◆ Anything you say now may be used against you at some point in the future. Using hate speech, expressing extreme or offensive views, trolling, etc is not a harmless activity. Victimising anyone online is an asshole's activity and likely to come back to bite you.

◆ Social media is not reality – it presents an idealised, simplified version of life. Avoid comparing yourself to anyone on the basis of their Instagram pics – the truth is likely to be much more complicated, and less filtered.

◆ Use privacy settings wisely. If you use multiple apps, keep them separate. Don't mingle personal with professional.

◆ Avoid over-sharing, particularly of suspect activities. You may be running for Prime Minister one day.

◆ Network, network, network – reach out to people you have met or have some connection with. You never know where opportunity might spring from.

◆ Don't spread yourself too thin, however. Less can be more – if you're struggling to update multiple platforms, cut it back to the essentials.

◆ Never use social media to complain about work, co-workers, managers, etc. This will come back to haunt you, possibly as early as tomorrow.

Your phone and you

We all now live our lives welded to a small device containing all the accumulated knowledge of man, and pictures of strangers' dinners. It is natural to want to know how many likes we got for that picture of a kitten eating a hotdog, but if the phone comes to dominate your life, there is a good argument to put it away. Dock it when you get home, and leave it there. It's good for your brain.

There are also some situations in which phone checking is a straight no, on grounds of flagrant rudeness:

◆ On a date. Obviously. Even if they are.

◆ At the till/cash desk. Checking your phone while someone asks you if you want a bag makes you look like an entitled asshole. Engage with the human.

◆ In a meeting, while someone else is talking. A quick way of showing you have somewhere more important to be, and aren't listening. In which case, why are you even here?

◆ While someone is trying to tell you something. Even a brief glance at an incoming message can make the person talking to you feel devalued.

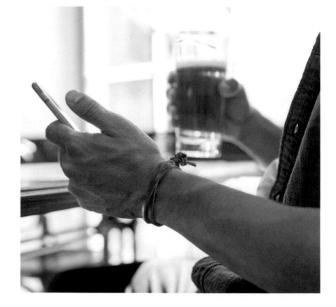

HOW TO
MANAGE A DINNER DATE

The first job when planning to take someone out to eat is choosing the venue. In the information age, there is no excuse for ignorance of the best place for the occasion. Use your imagination, read reviews and avoid chains or other unimaginative options.

If you don't know already, find out what your dinner-date likes – or more importantly, what they don't. They may prefer that you take the lead, and claim that 'anything is fine'. If that happens, feel free to take them at their word. If it is a romantic dinner, you'll want a certain amount of ambience, but don't make that the only consideration – an interesting menu will give you something to talk about, while candlelight and looming waiters can feel oppressive and make you self-conscious.

It isn't necessary to spend a lot of money to get a good meal, particularly if you live in or near a city with a variety of options (you will almost always get more bang for your culinary buck from international eateries – Thai, Japanese, etc). It helps to know something about the food you are eating, so if you have a favourite cuisine, let your choice demonstrate your knowledge and if it is obscure, be helpful with how to order and eat it – just avoid being a mansplaining bore. If you can, do a recce. Booking in person also allows you to check the ambience/dress code.

Rules for the night

- Wait for your date to sit before sitting.
- On a date, park your phone on silent and leave it face down or in your pocket. DO NOT TOUCH IT. Really.
- Let your date choose what they want first. If you know the menu, or think you can help, ask if you can assist.
- Before ordering drinks, ask if they have a preference. There's no rule that says it has to be wine, and a cocktail at the start can loosen things up nicely. If it is wine, establish what they like, and whether it is to be white or red based on what you are eating.
- Remember the purpose of you being offered a taste of wine before it is poured is solely to check whether it is spoiled, not to ask for your feedback.
- Mind your table manners. Napkins go on your lap, not tucked into your shirt. Cutlery skills matter in fine dining: cutlery is used from the outside in, and don't scoop food with the fork – instead push it on to the tines with the knife.
- Eat slooowly – do not gobble, or talk with food in your mouth. Maintain eye contact, and conversation. Avoid ordering food that is difficult to manage gracefully.

- Be polite and friendly to the waiting staff – rudeness reflects badly on you.
- If you need to go to the toilet, use an 'excuse me' and if you take your phone with you do not use it to post anything – such as details of how the date is progressing.
- Do not be embarrassed or overawed by the fanciness of the restaurant. They are selling food, and you are paying for it. You are the customer here.
- If something is wrong with the food, the drink or the experience, you are entitled to complain. Your companion may appreciate you doing this on their behalf, but don't steam in there without checking. Don't get angry or be rude – just calmly point out what is wrong, and what you want done about it.
- If you asked someone out, you are paying. This is not dependant on how the evening went – you asked, you pay.
- Tipping depends on where you are, but be aware that in many places staff rely on tips to make a living wage. In some places, the service charge will have been automatically added – only decline to pay it if the service has been truly bad. If you tip in cash, there is more chance it will go directly to the server.

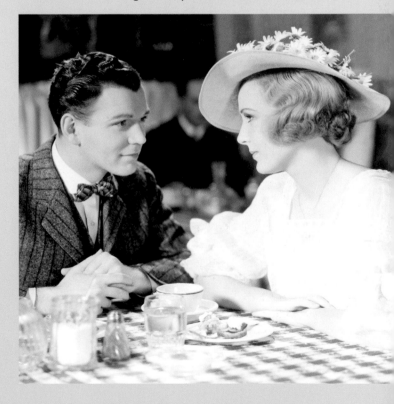

LIFE OF THE PARTY

Most of us are creatures of habit, and a man's downtime can be frittered away happily enough in the same old same old – bar, gaming, TV, repeat. If you want to get the most from life, step outside your norms and push yourself into new pursuits and pastimes. A rich life full of experiences is good for a man, and gives him something interesting to talk about. Taking on culture that's new to you has the power to expand your mind and help you grow.

Theatre

Live performance is not for everyone, but when you get the right play/cast/script, TV will feel like a pale imitation of the real thing. If you are new to theatre, look for something well reviewed that clicks with your taste, or scout around online for a random bargain. West End (London) or Broadway (New York) productions (or their equivalent in other countries) are the crème de la crème, but don't discount touring, regional versions. Look smart and dress comfortably. Don't be even slightly late – you won't be allowed in until the intermission. Be sure to turn off your phone, unless you want a room full of strangers staring angrily in your direction. Don't take in food.

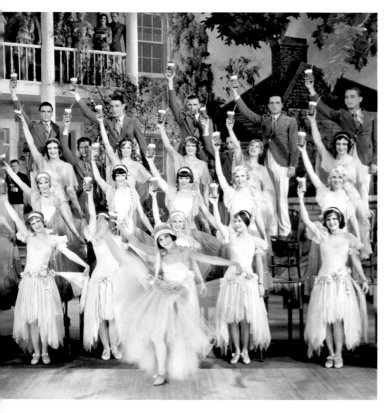

Cinema

Nothing beats the thrill of a darkened room full of strangers, a giant screen, and a sound system that will rattle your teeth. Treat yourself to a cinema experience you aren't used to – try IMAX for a new action movie, or an art house for foreign or classic films. Look out for special screenings, festivals and revivals, and treat yourself to an education in classic cinema. Old movies were meant to be seen in the cinema, without any distractions. A movie makes a great date night, it's true, but going to the cinema alone is one of life's great pleasures.

Gigs

Gigs offer excitement, unpredictability and a chance to dance like no one's watching (because they aren't). They are also great places to meet people – if you both like the band, you'll have at least one thing in common. Keep a watch on listings mags and fly-posters for local gigs, or get ambitious and Google dream gigs – the band you love may be playing somewhere you can reach with a cheap flight.

Festivals

Mud, sunshine, dancing in a field, random people, poor sanitation, great music, awful (sometimes wonderful) food, unexpected events. If that sounds like fun, you will already be familiar with the festival experience. There are enough on offer now that you can afford to be picky – shop around for a vibe or a line-up that you like the sound of. Some of the best festivals put the emphasis less on the big names and more on the good times and interesting venues.

Choose the team you are going with both for their fun factor and their ability to hold it together when someone has nicked your sleeping bag, or the tent has blown away. If you can't stand mud, choose a beach festival in Southern Europe, and if you can't stand sleeping on the ground, go upscale and get something incorporating glamping/a chalet. Pack carefully, and expect all plans to get lost along the way.

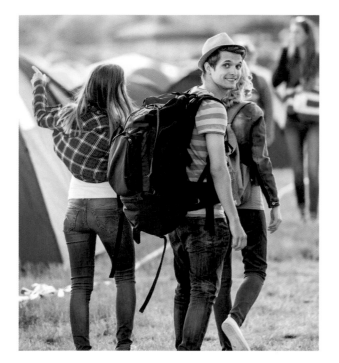

Sporting events

Nothing fills a man's life with more drama, anguish and delight than following a sport. Again, going against the grain will make life more interesting. If you support a big team, try taking in games at a lower division for an entirely different vibe – or at least a different pie/hotdog. Sport you have only watched on TV is a different proposition in the flesh. Treating yourself to a top-tier ticket to a premier event is not cheap, but it is likely to be highly memorable. Or do something altogether different, and watch a sport you aren't familiar with – odds are you will be able to watch local rugby, football/soccer, hockey, baseball, basketball, lacrosse, tiddlywinks teams for free, or at least on the cheap.

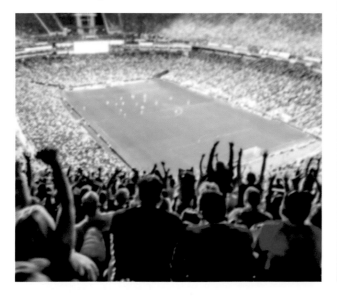

Take a trip

You don't need an excuse to go see somewhere different, but pegging your visit to an event makes for a memorable trip. The world is full of wild experiences – any of these are guaranteed to give you a story to tell…

◆ Palio di Siena, Siena, Italy. Demented, historical, bare-backed horse race through packed ancient piazza. A positively mediaeval vibe. July/August.
◆ La Tomatina, Valencia, Spain. Tomato-throwing festival. August.
◆ Nuit Blanche, Paris. Late-night arty high jinks in the city of lights. October.
◆ King's Day, Amsterdam, the Netherlands. No one parties like the Dutch. All over the Netherlands. Wear orange. April.
◆ Tour de France, France. If you are into cycling in a big way, joining a tour group and bringing your bike can sweep you up in the action. July.
◆ Monaco Grand Prix, Monaco. Formula 1 distilled to its essentials: noise, glamour, danger, ludicrously fast cars racing through tight streets at risk to themselves and the spectators. May.
◆ Calcio Storico, Florence, Italy. Violence parading as sport, in which teams of locals beat the living daylights out of each other in an ancient piazza. There's a ball involved somewhere. July.
◆ US Masters, Augusta, Georgia, USA. Heaven on earth for golf fans. April.
◆ El Clásico, Spain. Barcelona vs Real Madrid, a grudge match with a fevered atmosphere, reflecting long-established rivalries.
◆ Oktoberfest, Munich, Germany. The world's biggest beer party from mid-September to early October. Fill your boots with beer, sausages, deafening brass music, and more beer.
◆ Running of the Bulls, Pamplona, Spain. Who wouldn't want to risk life and limb legging it down narrow streets with angry cattle? July.

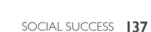

Rock the dance floor

Dancing is probably the most important skill a man can master, after listening. Dancing shows the world you have confidence, rhythm, balance and a sense of humour, but more importantly, there is no night that isn't made better with dancing. Having an indifferent time? Start dancing, and check back with me in an hour. It is also, coincidentally, the skill most directly connected to pulling, guaranteed to be more effective than any chat-up line.

Some men start from the assumption they can't/don't dance, and defend that position to the death. The only person suffering from this decision is you. Everyone can dance, and it is everyone's right to experience some of the fun that comes from it.

There are two approaches to learning to dance: winging it and taking classes. Assuming all you want to do at the outset is avoid embarrassment on a crowded dance floor, there is no risk in adopting the former approach, and lessening the shock of the nightclub or wedding disco with some light at-home practice. Remember, you aren't trying to win Mr Disco 1978, just to be able to blend in and enjoy a dance. You are looking to find your basic move, the core shuffle that will keep you going on the floor while you build confidence and think about adding a little ambition and a

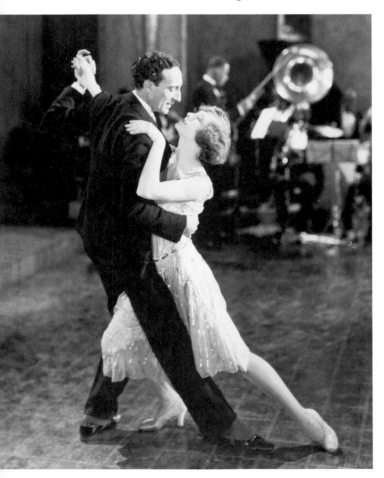

few moves. Draw the curtains and lock the door. You don't want to get busted. Put on a favourite track, ideally loud. Stand still, close your eyes and listen to the beat. Keeping your body relaxed, start to tap your feet and nod your head in time. Then dance.

All dancing involves is moving to the music, any way you please. If you feel stuck, and unnatural, start small. Sway to the beat. Let your arms move in time to the music, then your knees, shifting your weight from foot to foot, lifting the other off the ground a bit, as you swing your arms to the rhythm. Rotate your body slightly back and forth as you go. Yes it looks weird in a bedroom mirror, but on the dance floor no one will notice. Keep it going until it feels less unnatural. As you build confidence, get ambitious. Throw in small steps, stepping out and back in with alternating feet. Try stepping to the side, turning, bolder arm movements, pauses. Stay relaxed, hips and knees unlocked. Have fun.

And that's it. The best way to get used to dancing in a nightclub is to dance in a nightclub. Start with a favourite track you know well, and check the prevailing dance pace and style. If you are still self-conscious, wait until the floor gets full – no one will notice any awkwardness in your groove. Pretending you feel confident until you do is, as ever, a useful strategy. Focus on how it feels to you, not how it looks to others. Unless you are in a goth club, keep your head up and smile – looking like you are having a good time, and don't care if anyone is judging, is half the job.

The more you dance, the less weird it feels and the better the night gets. If you are drawn to clubs with a particular music policy and a particular accompanying dance, or a high standard – say, Northern Soul – then you'll need to do more homework. Watch videos, keep practising, look for people busting moves you can copy, or get lessons.

Dance classes

In general, dance classes may be better at preparing you for specific partner dances – such as salsa, jive or waltz – than they are about readying you for a generic dance-floor groove. The practice of learning steps can nevertheless give you techniques and moves that can be dropped on a dance floor, and lessons are unbeatable at building your confidence and stamina. Shop around for a class that interests you, and don't be afraid to take on a challenge. You don't need to bring a partner, but if you are in a couple (and at a more or less similar dancing/fitness level) it is a great way to bond and learn together.

Partner dancing

Dancing with a partner is easier if you've had a lesson or two, but you can fake it with a little effort. The man (that's you) is the leader, setting the pace and the direction. Job number one – maintain eye contact. Job number

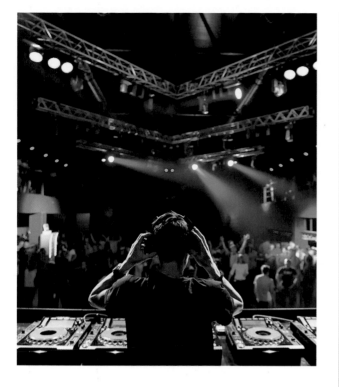

two – avoid stepping on their feet. If all you are doing is dancing near each other, just put yourself in front of them and dance as you feel it – you can copy each other's movements, but it doesn't have to be slavish.

When it gets to dancing in each other's arms, things get trickier. Line yourself up – not right in front, shoulder to shoulder, but slightly to the side. Put your right hand around their waist and hold it lightly at their lower back, palm flat, applying only the very lightest pressure. Hold your other arm out so as to take their hand, at about chest height (yours). Don't grip the hand too tightly, or interlock fingers – this isn't an arm wrestle. Leave a little gap between you – assuming it isn't yet a grinding situation.

Letting the music guide your rhythm, lead your partner in time. In ballroom dancing, the man leads and the woman follows, so picture yourself in the driving seat, setting the pace and showing her which way you want the dance to go. Use your hands to guide her – light pressure in the direction of travel will do it, as will shifting your weight where you aim to go. This is non-verbal communication, and if you work well together on the dance floor, you're going to be a good fit elsewhere.

Keep your steps small and simple – you should be lined up so you are not quite toe to toe, which helps you avoid stepping on your partner's. The most basic footwork is a box step, moving your feet through a square, the outside foot always doing the movement. Practise this, holding an imaginary partner, or get lessons – even if you don't use them for years there will come a day when you will be glad you have that knowledge tucked away somewhere.

Clubbing survival guide

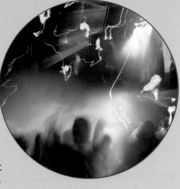

If you are already clubbing on a regular basis, you won't need advice on how to make the most out of your dance-floor good times. Others may want to challenge their assumption that the nightclub is not their idea of fun.

Plan ahead. Choose your night with care and in advance, rather than rocking up somewhere random because someone's mate fancies someone who might be there. Weekend nights may be more mobbed and less selective. Assemble your crew on the basis of both fun and reliability. Prepare yourself by eating a meal – it'll keep you going and stop things getting messier than you intended – and choose your outfit in advance. Make sure it's something appropriate to the night, which you can both look good and get sweaty in.

Pre-drinking will certainly make the night cheaper, and take the edge off any nerves, but turning up already smashed is somewhat pointless, since you could be anywhere. If you can't trust yourself, don't bring out all your cash/cards, or your expensive phone. Hiding cab/kebab money in a pocket or sock is a good strategy. Drink water.

Don't expect meaningful conversation – you wouldn't be able to hear it – but do have no shame when it comes to the dance floor. You came here to have a good time, not to look cool. Just listen to the rhythm and do what comes naturally. You will be surprised how quickly you start to lose any self-consciousness. You may think everyone is looking at you, but they aren't – they are too busy thinking about themselves. Speaking of which, don't bother taking pictures – the moment is more enjoyable when you don't record it. Fortune favours the brave – if you want to talk to or dance with someone, do. If it doesn't work, odds are they are unlikely to remember.

Most importantly, know when it is time to give it up and go home.

MODERN MANNERS

Manners and etiquette are constantly evolving, and what might be the correct thing to do according to the letter of the law may seem stiff and formal in the real world. A few years ago, men just didn't hug — now they embrace at the drop of a hat. In all questions of manners, use your best judgement.

Shaking hands

In British culture at least, the handshake is the almost universal starting point for greetings and goodbyes. Use it in most work scenarios, including when meeting someone for the first time, when seeing someone again after a while or when taking your leave of the person whose hand you shook on the way in. In some social situations it may feel a bit formal — and some men are content with a nod. Don't force it, and follow the lead of the person you are meeting.

Avoid extremes. Too many men seek to prove themselves by gripping their counterpart's hand like it was an opponent to be squashed into submission. This leaves an impression, but it's the wrong one — you will be remembered as a competitive, insecure man trying to one-up himself and score points in a test of strength.

The other side of the coin, and equally awful, is the limp rag — the hand passed over like a damp tea towel shows a disdain for the fellow shaker and leaves the lingering sense of someone who was not particularly keen to leave any impression at all.

Go for the middle ground. Ensure your hands are dry, for a start — this is why it is always worth drying your hands properly in the bathroom. Make eye contact as you extend your hand, and maintain it throughout, smiling. Repeating their name back to them — 'Nice to meet you, Simon' — ensures they know you are engaged (if there is any chance you may have met previously — settle for 'How are you?'). Let palm meet palm, and grip their hand — firmly, but not like you are trying to choke poultry. Shake from the elbow, not the shoulder — two goes, up and down, and disengage. Only go for a two-handed handshake if you know them well, and maybe want to express something — such as support in a hard time.

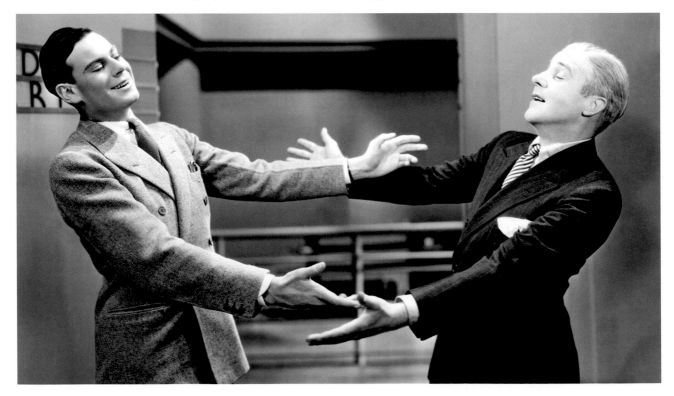

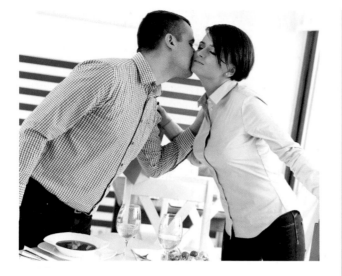

Kissing hello

Nothing represents the modern manners minefield better than the kiss. There is no reliable hard rule on precisely when and where someone might go for a kiss – but in the UK it is generally reserved for friends and close acquaintances. Those who live elsewhere, identify as continental or work in the arts, may have a different view. Unless you want to be perceived as a bit over-eager, your best strategy is to err on the side of caution, and watch for the signals that suggest someone might welcome a cheek kiss. Unless you know, or strongly suspect they are kissers, an outstretched hand is a safer bet.

This isn't so much a kiss as an imitation of one, a very light brushing of the cheek or the lip area to their cheek, no sound effects required and no real kissy contact either. In the UK, one cheek is common. If meeting a European, assume they will go for alternating cheeks – unless they are from Switzerland, where three kisses is the norm.

Hugging it out

Like the kiss, the hug is in a grey area, as men transition from a world in which an occasional hearty handshake was as physically affectionate as a chap got. Blame globalisation, Hollywood or getting in touch with our feelings – the unexpected hug is now a clear and present danger. Worse, there is no real rule on when, where or who to hug, leaving a man not quite sure where he stands.

Err on the side of caution. The risk that someone might think you are crossing a boundary, or making a pass, is real, and on balance the charge of inappropriate behaviour is probably worse than the chance they will think you stand-offish. In general, don't initiate a hug unless you are fairly certain it is a mutual impulse. Save it for old friends, close and affectionate family members, and loved ones – or for others in special circumstances where you feel moved to display affection, such as when they receive good news.

Being a gentleman

Etiquette can vary according to where you are, but these general rules always apply:

Always:
◆ hold the door for the person coming in behind you
◆ allow the person you're with to enter first/sit down first/order first
◆ be quick to give up your seat for anyone who might need it more than you
◆ be polite and friendly to people serving you – if they ask how you are return the compliment.

Never:
◆ manspread, keep your knees together and your feet/bag off the seat
◆ mansplain (you know what that is, right? It's when a man explains a concept to someone at great length when the person they are addressing is already familiar… oh, I see what you've done here…)
◆ on public transport: eat smelly food; conduct loud personal calls; listen to crap music on crap headphones super loud
◆ start eating before others have been served unless they say you can
◆ dump someone by text (there may be an exception for when they are clearly and inarguably in the wrong, *eg* you caught them cheating)
◆ brag about conquests, sexual or otherwise.

However, be ready for someone else to initiate it, and unless it is truly unwelcome, don't be the uptight guy, the man who doesn't know how to deal with it. Roll with it, and hug right back. If you want to stick in a back clap or two, go for it – just not one of those stiff claps some men do in the hope it makes the whole thing seem less touchy feely.

For bro-to-bro interactions, there is a decent compromise – the clasped-hand shoulder bump, in which a handshake morphs into a quick coming together of torsos and a slap on the back from the free hand. This lacks the commitment of the full hug, so works as a substitute – but you both have to be on the same page, or it may get awkward. Save it for guys you know well.

A note of caution – for colleagues, managers or people you manage there are very, very good reasons for keeping it formal. A handshake is hard to misunderstand.

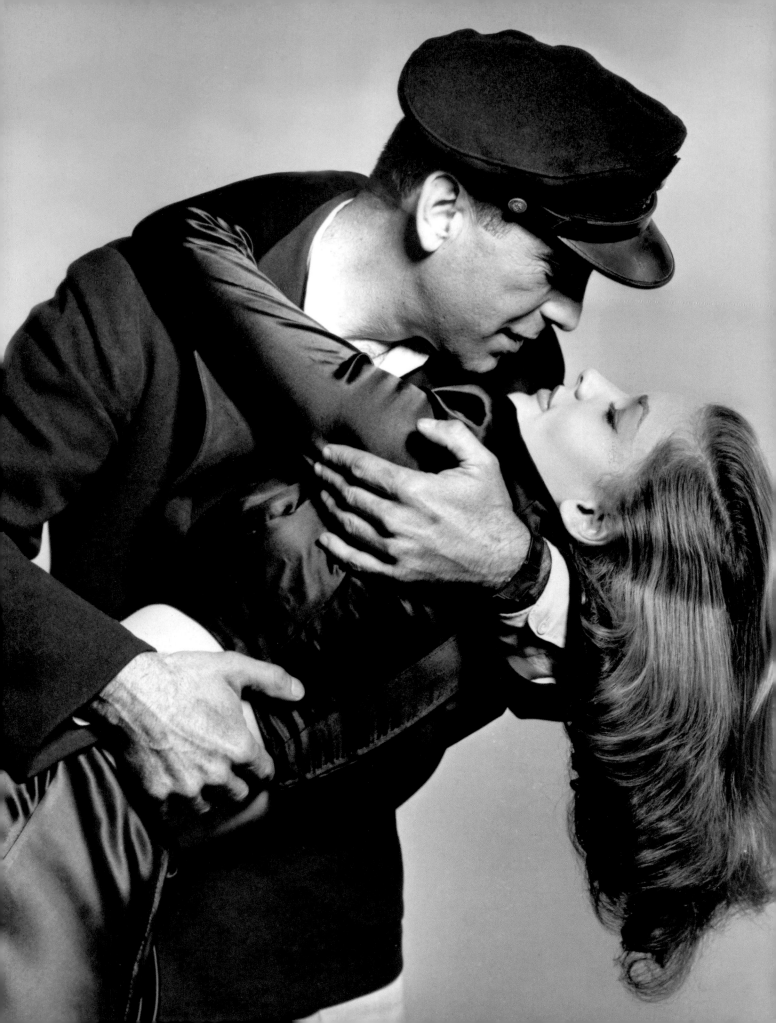

CHAPTER 6

DATING AND RELATIONSHIPS

No man is an island, and most of us will struggle to feel complete without some kind of meaningful relationship. Technology may have altered how we meet prospective partners, but it can't change the ground rules entirely. It is still the case that any man who wants love needs to know how to make the most of himself, present his best image to the world, and own the communication skills necessary for building a real relationship. Whether he is looking for The One, or the one for tonight.

ONLINE DATING

Internet dating is the cold hard reality of our era. Once upon a time a man was limited in whom he could meet, and where – now a whole wide world of prospective partners is within reach. It's an exciting development in theory, but fraught with pitfalls.

There is no rule that says as a single man you must be out there online. Of course you can just stick to your existing social media habits, and it's entirely possible you will meet people that way. If you do choose internet dating, which site/app you choose depends on who you want to meet and why. If all you are looking for is a casual hook-up, there's an app for that. Many apps in fact.

Hook-up apps

Some guys may have less interest in love, and more in booty. If that's you, make your interests clear and only use those sites that find you someone for tonight. Specifying what you are after (everyone knows what 'casual, short-term fun' means) offers less risk that anyone will look to you for love.

The hook-up world can be a mercenary, brutal business but it suits some people, particularly those with thick skins, who don't mind rejecting (and being rejected back) for the most shallow of reasons. Choose your photos accordingly. Before you commit to a hotel-room assignation, give yourself the chance to check each other against those flattering photos. Keep it safe (let a friend know where you are going and who you are meeting, wear a condom) and

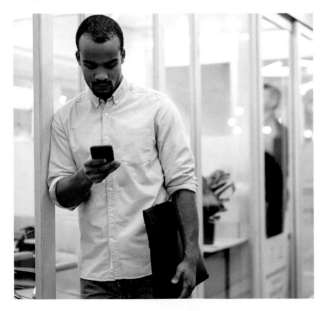

keep it honest (getting into a thing with someone who has a partner may lead to more trouble than you can imagine).

Choosing a dating site

If you are after something serious, or are at least open to the idea, then look for the site or app that is most likely to deliver it. Some attract a particular type – those with liberal political views, or gym bunnies – which may help narrow it down. Don't be afraid to go against what you think is your type, or assume that only someone into the same stuff as you could possibly make a good match. If you prefer the less-pressured experience of safety in numbers, some sites are more about social connections and group hang-outs. For the practical-minded you can go for apps that prioritise location – though these are often less about love and more about sex.

Building a profile

When you've chosen a site that fits your idea of who you are after, build a profile. Honesty is the best policy – however, remember this is a sales pitch, so don't linger on the negatives. Think strategically and market yourself to your target audience. Who are you aiming for, and what is likely to capture their interest? Think about what makes you different, a good companion, a love interest. Steer clear of clichés and bland statements. 'I like watching TV' – yeah, me too, but so what? Take time, and use your skills and personality. Write something that is you, that has your humour in it, and reflects your outlook. Look at the profiles that attracted you, and think about why they worked.

Marketing yourself doesn't mean using naked dishonesty. Hiding something about yourself that will be immediately obvious in real life is not the greatest approach. It shows you to be a liar about the little things, such as whether you have hair, or are recently divorced. Use humour, and a direct approach. Women (and men) appreciate a man who is down with his own self, who has the confidence to admit to imperfections and laugh at his own follies.

There is a fine line to be struck between over-sharing and underplaying it. A bit of mystery is no bad thing, but don't overdo it. Too much information is always a bad thing – not only does it risk your privacy, it can be a turn-off, particularly if you give off the desperate or sad vibe. That is the quickest way to guarantee they run for the hills, so no self-pity, unless it is the wry and funny kind. Similarly, walk a middle line with confidence. Watch for too much modesty (if you say you are nothing special, expect people to agree) but don't come across as cocky (people who brag are usually concealing insecurity).

Selecting profile pics

You know that picture in which you look pretty handsome, actually, and are doing something interesting, such as nursing a wounded koala or helping orphans dig a well? That one. Find a picture that shows you in a good light, doing something you love.

Don't:

◆ Use an image that is a total lie, intentionally concealing something, or carefully cropped to cut something or someone out.
◆ Upload several posed solo selfies. This indicates vanity – instead, pictures of you with friends and family show your social side.
◆ Use an extreme close-up – show at least part of your body, or they may wonder why you haven't.
◆ Use a picture that is really hilarious but not flattering – remember, this is marketing.

Do:

◆ Go for natural rather than posed – get someone to snap you doing something in real life. Keep it relaxed.
◆ Wear clothes. Wear good clothes – look approachable but well groomed. And not naked.

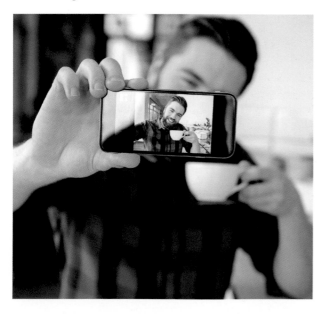

Online dating fails

◆ Be too keen. Rushing it, or coming across as desperate, is going to drop you points. You don't need to game play, but neither should you be looking to seal the deal before you've met. Be honest, but be cool.
◆ Be coy. If you like someone, reach out – don't wait for them to come to you.
◆ Linger in pen pal cyberspace, swapping messages with someone for weeks. If it looks like a good fit, do something, or get off the pot.
◆ Expect the moon on the stick. This is real life – some people you won't fancy, and some won't fancy you.
◆ Argue with rejection. Take 'no' for an answer first time, every time. Ditto silence, which is also 'no'.
◆ Offer unsolicited negative feedback – 'your feet are too big' helps no one.

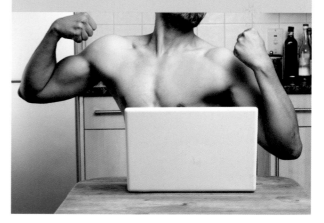

◆ Use good lighting – outdoors is best, and use a friend to hold the camera.
◆ Add more than one photo.
◆ Include an interesting or memorable setting or backdrop. It helps someone start a conversation ('Hey, I see you like helping wounded koalas dig wells for orphans – me too!').

Would like to meet

Don't assume you know perfectly well what you need in life or love, and that only a 6ft+ Nordic blonde who likes track cycling could possibly be a good match. If there are some real non-negotiables (if you just can't stand to date any more lingerie models) be upfront with it. Otherwise, keep the 'looking for' section open and flexible, and do not make it look like you are shopping for a car. Those 'must haves' are a turn-off, even for those lucky people who tick your long list of boxes.

MEETING PEOPLE IRL

In theory, online dating is the most efficient way of giving you maximum chances to pull/find a life partner. However, theory doesn't always translate into practice, and the truth is, online isn't for everyone. For one thing, there is no algorithm that will tell you if you have chemistry with someone. For some, the data-driven approach feels mechanical and forced, lacking in excitement, romance, humour.

If online dating isn't delivering, or you suspect there is more to life than endless swiping, delete the app and get back into reality.

If it has been a while, expect it to feel a little weird at first. As we have adjusted our lives to the constant presence of mobile technologies and social media, we have begun to lose basic human skills. There's more on the line when you approach someone in the real world, more risk than pinging an emoticon to a stranger. The good news is that the thrill is also greater. Because risk and reward go hand in hand, and sweaty palms, a thumping heart and a sick stomach are the world's way of letting you know you are truly alive.

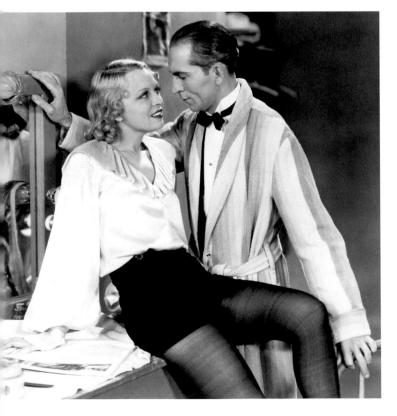

Where to meet people

If you lift your head from your phone, you will notice the world is full of people, a number of whom are attractive and interesting. Your daily life will bring you into contact with some of them, which is a good place to start. There's your commute, your workplace, your neighbourhood, your favourite cafe, the gym, the pub. It's true there's a risk involved in asking out someone you see every day, and a rebuff may mean some embarrassment later on, but it may be worth taking that chance anyway.

Tread carefully at work, where proximity can build closeness but which might be fraught with tensions and employment law. Friends of friends offer a very good chance of a relationship – you already have people in common, which is a good place to start, and may point to more shared interests, plus you can get some background on them with little effort. If you are interested and have a mutual friend, engineer something – a group drink or similar. Events (most of all weddings) are tried-and-tested venues for the bachelor to meet singles connected to him through friends or family.

You can't beat meeting someone through a shared passion. If you haven't currently got an interesting pursuit that might expose you to romance, it's easy enough to find one. Go to dance classes, sign up for book clubs, go to gigs, and you will run across people who like at least some of the same things as you. Shared interests are not, of course, a guarantee of love or lust – but they are a damn good place to start.

No such thing as 'out of your league'

Many guys hesitate to approach someone who seems too good for them – limiting the chances available to them and reinforcing their own insecurities. Start from the assumption that no one is out of your league, ever. Yes, extraordinarily beautiful people may be aware they are extraordinarily beautiful … but then again, they may have insecurities too, among them a fear that people only like them for their looks. Engaging their mind, and looking for the person behind the perfect facade may work for both of you. Fearlessness builds confidence – if you truly believe there is no good reason not to ask out a Nobel-prize-winning model on a date, that sense of your own limitlessness will transmit itself to them and the world at large.

Fortune favours the brave. If you see someone you think you would like to get to know, you only have to do one thing – speak. Open your mouth, and let words come out. About anything. 'Hello' will do. Avoid cheesy or prepared lines – these reveal you to be a would-be player, lacking character and charm. Instead just break the ice, and see what happens. Be interested, ask questions, be charming, but above all, be yourself.

Your aim is another meeting, but let's be clear – you are looking for more than a friend. It's a date, make sure there is no misunderstanding on that point. Ask for a number, and don't wait days to call it.

Have a suggestion in mind – not just 'Let's hang out' but something more interesting. Dinner is fine, if uninspired, a drink may be a little lighter, a coffee lighter still. Use your imagination, and keep your eyes and ears open for ideas. If you're lucky enough to be approached by someone, smile, be gracious, and consider saying yes. It's only a date.

Playing the game

Countless books have been sold to guys on the basis that relations with wo/men can be reduced to a series of tactics designed to ensure you get to sleep with them and move on. And the truth is, some of them work. However, if you go down that path, don't expect happiness at the end of it. All such games require deception and manipulation, treating someone as an object to be pursued, rather than a person in their own right. For anyone with a conscience, the satisfaction gained from any 'victory' gained by misrepresenting yourself or your interest in them will feel hollow. If it doesn't, and you are happy to play the bastard, know that one day you too will be played.

Don't game play – everyone has read the advice on waiting three days, and everyone knows when a player is playing. Better to go with your gut and call when seems right (subject to some common sense about not pestering, or appearing too cool to care). If you aren't pretending to be anything other than what you are, you won't have to remember any lies, and will have the reward of being appreciated for being your own self. This is the strategy of no strategy, and it works.

Handling rejection

The first rule of rejection is to recognise it. If the object of your affections is ignoring your interest, or offering short,

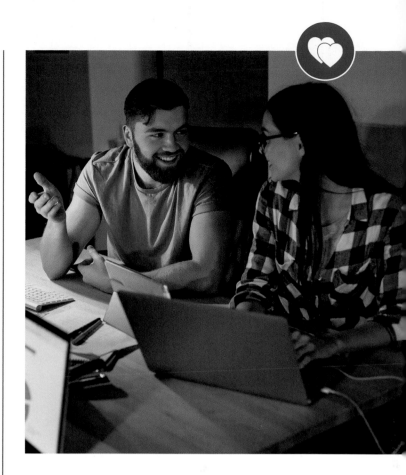

polite responses without warmth, assume that's a no. Leave it there. Your charm is not going to bring them round – and to continue to pursue someone who isn't into you is creepy.

Nothing ventured, nothing gained – if you strike out, chalk it up to experience and let it go. You thought it might work, it didn't, c'est la vie – at least you had the nerve to find out. Don't let it bring you down, and if it does, commiserate with friends.

Don't hit on someone when

◆ they are doing something sweaty in the gym
◆ they quite clearly wish to be left alone – wearing headphones and/or reading a book means 'do not disturb'
◆ they work for you
◆ they are the person who makes your coffee every day – if the approach doesn't work, you're probably going to have to go somewhere else, and coffee is very important
◆ they have mentioned their partner – this is generally a clue to leave it (unless they said it in a 'my boyfriend is so dull, not like you' kind of way)
◆ they say no, or act disinterested.

FIRST DATES, SECOND DATES

A first date is enormously important … but you can't let it show. This is you, in the shop window. You will need to project confidence, charm, warmth and any other characteristics that might make your new date want to come back for more. Assuming that's what you want. If it is, you will need an attitude and a plan. And deodorant.

Venue

Offering to go 'wherever you like' will tick none of your date's boxes. This is not a moment for the politely passive approach. Demonstrate confidence and make a choice, but don't insist on it. You are putting up a suggestion for approval, and while you want to be self-assured, you don't want to seem inflexible or bossy.

In an ideal world, a first date will reflect something about your date and/or your shared interests – if you've been able to establish them. In situations where you don't have much to go on, there are two choices: something entirely new or something safe, which is already your kind of thing. For the former, the bond that can form as you try new experiences can work serious magic if the chemistry is right, but be

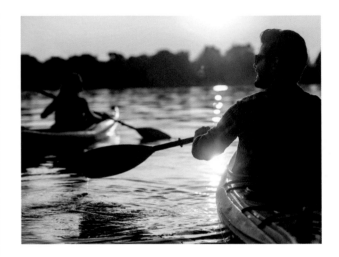

aware you risk showing incompetence. Be prepared to laugh at yourself if you aren't as good at pottery as you thought you might be. If you go for option b, you have the advantage of appearing confident and sure of yourself. However, make sure it is something that your date might conceivably enjoy. Don't drop them in at the deep end of your tastes – if you don't know their views on kung-fu movies, an all-night marathon is not the place to find out. This is not a test for them to pass, but a chance for you to connect, and challenge your assumptions about what and who you want. You may believe you could only find love with someone who enjoys octopus sashimi and long walks in the rain, but you may be wrong.

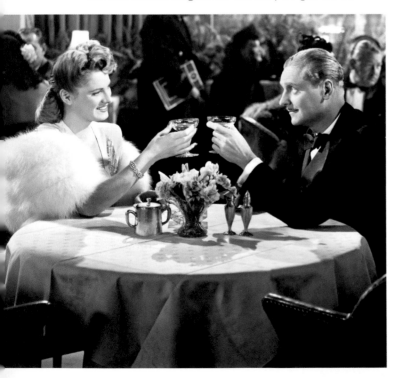

'Men always want to be a woman's first love – women like to be a man's last romance'
Oscar Wilde

DATE IDEAS

Movies

The first-date option of choice for a hundred years or so, this allows you to sit in quiet companionship and share a cultural experience. On the upside, you have something to talk about afterwards but it won't actually help you to get to know them. Choose the film with great, great care – 'someone I know' once took a first date to a Japanese art film that turned out to be 120 minutes of hard-core sex. Art-house cinemas offer sofa seats, wine in glasses, good snacks and interesting films – that elevate the experience. Meet for a drink beforehand to say hello first.

Dinner

This is where you get to demonstrate your taste and sophistication. However, and this is important, don't let your drive to impress overwhelm your better instincts. This is also about an experience your date can enjoy, and if they aren't particularly adventurous, exploring vegan Peruvian wholefoods may not be the best idea. Remember – if you invited, you pay, however the evening goes – so don't go more expensive than you can afford.

Drinks

Once upon a time, going for a drink meant finding the least sticky corner of a dingy pub. Now, your choice is enormous. Choose a venue based on how formal/fancy you want the evening to be. If you are putting on a display of sophistication, and can afford it, a cocktail bar is the way to go. If the date feels less formal then a good pub is fine – provided it is on the upscale end of the spectrum.

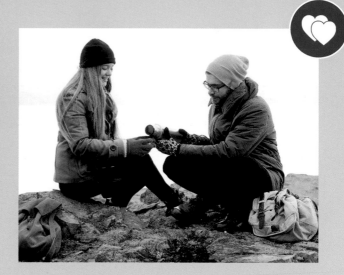

Activities

A date that takes both of you out of your comfort zone will win you points for creativity, provided you choose carefully. Be sure your date is fully forewarned of what is involved though. No woman will be happy to find she is expected to hike across a muddy field in heels.

◆ An art exhibition allows you to demonstrate your cultural nous (read up on the artists before you get there) while taking a companionable stroll.
◆ A dance class is a fun shortcut to testing out your chemistry – this works best if you are at the same level.
◆ Bowling engages light competition, involves beer if desired, and gives you a distraction to focus on.
◆ Afternoon tea is a neat twist on going for coffee, and more charming/light than a full-on dinner.
◆ A picnic is a good way to demonstrate your culinary skills, plus it is cheap. Bring drinks, a blanket, and choose the location well in advance.
◆ Use your imagination: climbing, cycling, hiking…

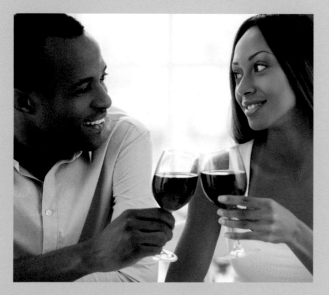

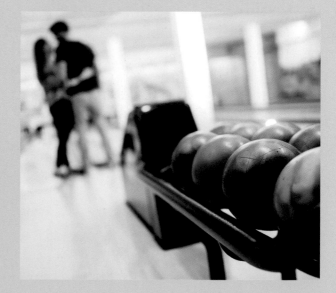

Secrets of a successful first date

Because different people have different needs, there is no magic formula, no skeleton key to unlock every heart. That said, a few good habits will give you the edge – because the truth is, there are many useless men out there, and fulfilling these most basic of requirements will give you an advantage over them.

◆ Dress well. You are going to be judged. The formality will depend on the venue, but at the very least clad yourself in a manner flattering to your figure that is also reasonably smart and clean. Nails, hair, breath, socks, fragrance – everything matters.

◆ Get there first, even if it means being really early.

◆ Ask questions. Not like they're in a job interview, instead express a genuine curiosity about them and their personality – enough that you keep the focus on them, rather than yourself. Listen. Properly. This is really really important.

◆ Smile. Make it apparent you are enjoying their company. Laugh when they tell a joke, convincingly. If you are having a good time, tell them. But…

◆ Be cool. Being openly interested in someone is appealing. Being so blown away by them that you keep telling them you are blown away by them makes you look intense/desperate.

◆ Do not talk about your exes, or anything that makes you bitter and angry. Focus instead on things you love or are proud of.

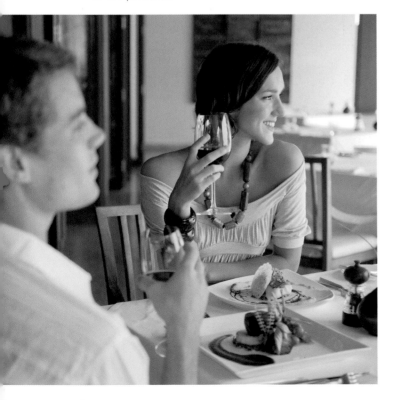

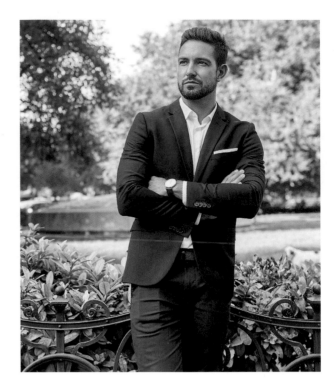

How to decline a second date

Some combinations are just not meant to be, and you may have realised moments after sitting down that your date for the evening is not your idea of a good time. Before you commit yourself to that call, slow down and check any assumptions you are bringing to the table – such as unfeasible standards. If this sounds like you, stop and ask yourself why no one is ever quite right, and consider spending more time with Ms Not Quite until you are sure your first instincts are the right ones. Or take a break from dating.

If it's a straight no, extricate yourself as cleanly and quickly as possible while causing the least amount of damage. You haven't committed to anything, so in theory that should be straightforward – however, remember that rejection can sting. Least said, soonest mended – don't offer unsolicited negative feedback, but be ready to politely decline any follow-up approach you might get. Keep it short and civil, and remember it's hard to argue against feelings. You don't feel ready for a relationship, you're not over your ex, there wasn't a spark, you are going to be spending time on your own.

When there is some legitimate expectation for more from the other side, disappearing without warning or a word of explanation is an asshole's trick – it gets you out of there, but leaves pain in your wake. Be ready for embarrassment if you ever meet again. Better to rip off the plaster/Bandaid politely but quickly – and hope anyone who feels this way towards you treats you with the same respect.

HOW TO
GUARANTEE A SECOND DATE

If you know you want to see them again, start by accepting that despite what is implied above, there can be no guarantee, ever. Sometimes you want to date people who don't want to date you, and sometimes it works the other way round. That's life, and there is nothing to be gained from mooching about, wondering what you did wrong. Particularly because you may very well have done absolutely nothing wrong. You don't know this person well enough to be familiar with what kind of stuff may be going on in their head/heart, or what their personal history may be.

Unless they volunteer the information, you just have to not know, and be fine with that. Reasons for rejection don't always make sense, and don't necessarily say anything bad or insightful about you. So whatever, accept it, and if they volunteer a clue for your future conduct in their rejection (eg 'I only date men who brush their teeth') take it and move on.

NB Some men go insane about being brushed off, demonstrating an inflated sense of their own worth and a deep insecurity. Don't be the guy who gives the rest of us a bad name with bitchy tweeting, name calling and other acts of outrage.

If you are on the first date and already fairly sure you want more, reflect on the good news: they said yes once,

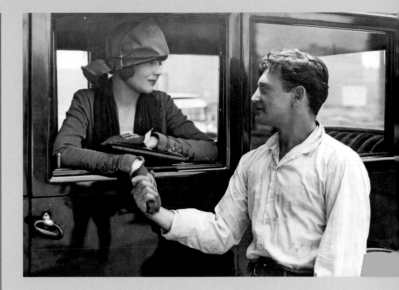

so you are already way ahead of the game. Cling on to that fact, and let it give you some confidence.

Look back on the marketing exercise. What do you know about what they want, and can you tick those boxes? Keep your eyes and ears open for clues – about what they don't like, as much as what they do. Be yourself, but be mindful of their wants and needs. Romance is a dance, in which you must read the clues of your partner. If s/he tells you s/he can't abide men who are obsessed with sport, do not mention your season ticket.

- ◆ Don't try too hard. Let the fact you are interesting, cool, warm, funny and not insane be apparent from what you say and how you act.

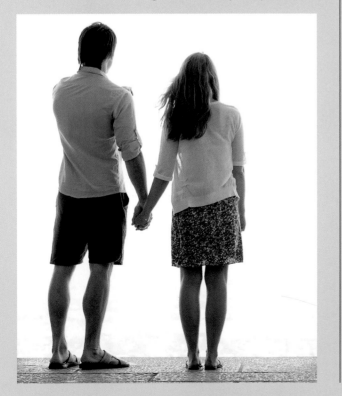

'Integrity is not a conditional word. It doesn't blow in the wind or change with the weather. It is your inner image of yourself, and if you look in there and see a man who won't cheat, then you know he never will'
John D Macdonald

BOYFRIEND MATERIAL

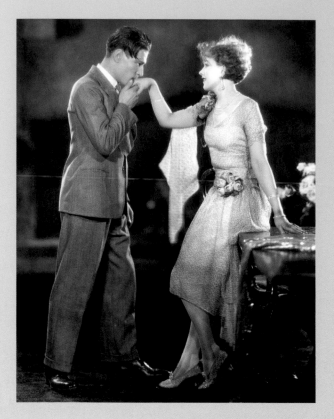

A man has to accept he is going to be judged, often and harshly. You will have been reviewed from top to toe by your date in a matter of moments. Before you've taken your coat off, s/he has a fair idea of whether this is a 'yes' or a 'no'. By the second drink, s/he's decided you're a second date. Or not. By the time the bill comes, s/he'd be able to tell a friend with some degree of confidence whether you are/are not Boyfriend Material.

A man with potential

It isn't a good idea to generalise about people and their needs based on their gender. What women want from a man could fill a very large book, one as infinite as the personalities, dreams and desires of womankind. While you can't draft a one-size-fits-all checklist, you can certainly meet a few basic criteria that mark you out as a man with potential, possessing the qualities a modern man is expected to bring to the table.

Straight men may imagine that a man looking for a man will have an easier time of it, which should get a hollow laugh from any gay guy. The gay world is as fraught with confusion as the straight. It's no easier to generalise about what a man might look for in a partner than it is a woman, but these broad guidelines should help maximise your chances.

Genes

From a strictly biological point of view, anyone looking for a man for the purposes of reproducing may consider your genetic profile – your manly jaw, shiny eyes, glossy mane, wet nose. There's not much you can do about your genes, so concentrate instead on what you do with what you've got – how you carry yourself, and transmit information about what kind of partner you would be.

Confidence

A strong, tangible manifestation of your belief in yourself is very attractive. Not cockiness, but the sense you are comfortable in your own skin (and clothes), the ability to remain relaxed in the face of pressure and to not spend too much time worrying about what others think of you. A confident man can hold a conversation with anyone, laugh at himself, and is happy to let others talk. He doesn't boast or bully, and people warm to him because he isn't looking to them for approval or feeling the need to compete. If you don't feel that way naturally, fake it.

Presentation

Turning up showered and shaved and dressed with due care and attention to detail sends out several powerful signals. It enhances whatever gifts nature gave you and shows you were prepared to make an effort. Most of all, it advertises the fact you are capable of looking after yourself – and therefore someone else, too.

Charm

An offshoot of confidence, charm is a magical quality that makes people warm to you. You can't manufacture it, but you can tip the odds in your favour. Smile (including with your eyes), use humour, make people feel important and interesting. Be happy to meet strangers, and let it show – use their name, shake their hand, make eye contact, remember something about them. Be empathetic ('How did that make you feel?') instead of competitive ('Oh yeah, I've done that') and be ready to laugh at yourself.

Faithfulness

Your ability to commit to one sexual partner at a time ticks an ancient biological imperative box, demonstrating you are likely to be present during the childhood of any offspring. In a modern context, your skill at keeping it in your pants is more straightforward – it demonstrates you are not an asshole and are mature enough to recognise that knocking boots with someone else is not cool. The belief that infidelity is sexy is wrong.

Ambition

The fact some people find ambition attractive doesn't necessarily mean they are interested in your annual salary. It is more likely that they find someone who is interested, engaged and driven more fun to be with than someone happy to sit on their arse and let life do to them whatever it wants. Have a passion, have a desire, and pursue it. It doesn't have to be to do with your career, but it does have to be to do with you. And don't be afraid to let your passion show – it's a turn-on.

GSOH

Having a sense of humour doesn't mean you can do word-perfect impressions of stand-up routines, so don't attempt to drop these in on a first date. Humour means you can laugh at yourself, the world, and someone else's jokes, that you have a sense of the absurdities of life and don't take it all too seriously – particularly yourself.

Reliability

Say what you are going to do, and do it. Turn up on time, sober, holding the thing you were supposed to bring. Remember birthdays, anniversaries, significant dates. We are all of us navigating a difficult and uncertain world, and we need a partner we can count on. A potential significant other is not going to talk commitment with a man who can't commit to the little things.

Romance

Setting out to woo shows you are sensitive, appropriately impassioned and confident. You don't need a white stallion – well-timed flowers, thoughtful gifts and a little dramatic flourish will go a long way. NB Overdoing it in the early days, or when they aren't actually that interested yet, may be oppressive – watch for signs that your grand gesture will go down well before you hire the Eiffel Tower.

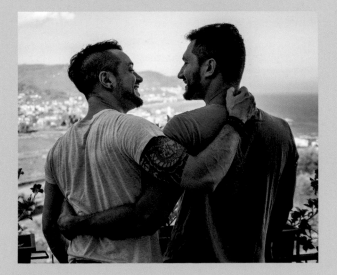

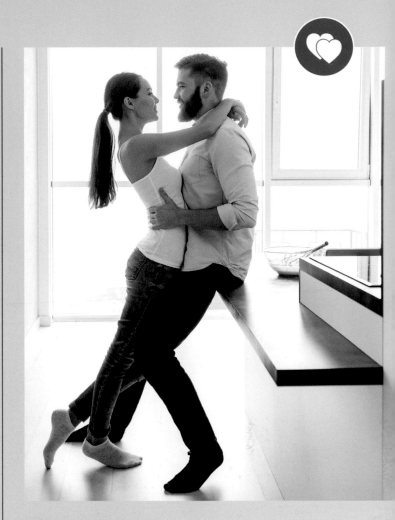

Dadness (potential)

Demonstrating the skills of fatherhood brings us back to biological imperatives. It may be way too early to actually contemplate parenting together, but that doesn't mean the concept of it might not enter into the equation, on some deep level. The qualities that will make you a good dad are impressive in their own right – maturity, patience, kindness. Those aren't the kind of 'manly' virtues ad companies use to sell razors, but they are profoundly sexy nonetheless.

Sex

Yep. You need to deliver consistent and high-quality bed-based experiences, or the ship won't float. Get used to being the giver – find out what your partner likes, and oblige. 'Good in bed' does not mean pounding away for hours like a rabbit on steroids – it means you can learn to read their needs and anticipate them, to be gentle when appropriate and strong when that's what's called for. If you don't know how to give a wo/man (actually, this wo/man) an orgasm, learn. Patience and sensitivity will get you further than hard gym hours. Above all, let your partner know it is them you want, not sex with whoever is available.

READING THE SIGNS

When love and sex moved from real life on to a screen, a whole new world of communication developed. Instant, but painfully easy to misunderstand. A conversation in person is full of visual cues that help you to understand what the other person is saying. A conversation online or by text is a guessing game, where what one person thinks is a pretty clear message can mean nothing to the person receiving it.

Emoji blues

There's no guarantee that what a person says by text, email or on an app can be translated into something that makes sense – because sometimes, people don't actually know what they are trying to say. There are also those who practise deliberate vagueness, people who intentionally send a mixed message, and a host of other communication nightmares that will mess with your head – often because that is what they have been designed to do.

People have different styles, so don't take the interpretations opposite too literally. Maybe you didn't get any kisses back because her phone doesn't have an 'X' button. Right. That's probably it.

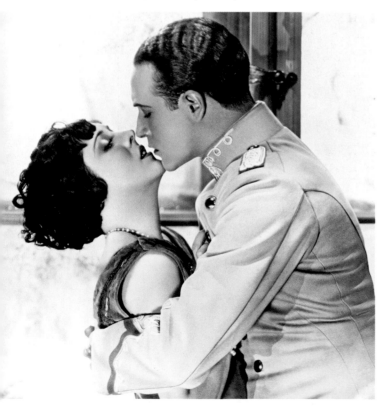

Love comms

If you want to have a significant discussion, do it in person. If it's time to step the relationship up a gear, or move on, if you want to start seeing more of them, or more of other people, make it face to face. Nothing gets missed and no one goes away wondering what they just agreed to. If you can't do it in person, the phone call is a distant second best.

Whatever the message, keep it super clear and hard to misunderstand, unless you have damn good reason to be vague. Men who send messages that could be read either way can be infuriating. Which might not put someone off, but that's not a good reason to be woolly. If you are into someone, practise mirroring instead – send messages that match theirs in terms of length and affection/flirtiness.

Do not volunteer to send a picture of your penis to anyone. Odds are that your little gentleman is more interesting to you than them, and once it's out there, it's not coming back.

The letter is the height of romance – if you can remember how to use a pen, and have something to say that you really want to hit home, buy good paper and a stamp and write a letter.

How to dump someone

There is no other acceptable way to let someone go other than in person, unless the fling was so light – on both sides – that a formal ending would be disproportionate, or someone got busted for a major foul, such as cheating. Tread carefully with separation and be aware that sometimes people aren't on the same page. What seemed like a booty call to you may have felt different to the owner of the booty in question – or vice versa.

Don't prevaricate. If you have convinced yourself this is the right thing to do, don't wait and wait, or misbehave in the hope they notice and dump you first. Disappearing with no explanation is about the worst thing you can do. If you haven't decided, then talk it through – it might be

What messages really mean

Message	Meaning
You swapped numbers, they texted first.	Into you. Probably. If you feel the same way, don't play it cool. Swift response.
You send three kisses. They send one.	Not that into you. Maybe.
You send one kiss. They send three.	Into you.
Three-day delay in response.	Unless accompanied by a very good excuse, not that into you. OR has read a book on how to play a man.
You send a super-long message. Theirs is short.	Not that into you. Or very busy. If it keeps happening, it's the first.
Sexy language.	Super into you, or at least your body. Let's get it on.
Please send dick pic ASAP	Hi. I'm a blackmailer, based out of Estonia. That picture of me is scanned from a lingerie catalogue. Prepare to see your penis exposed online.
Silence	Nah. Not happening.
Hey. What r u up to? X	(08:00–19:00): I like you. Let's hang out. (19:00–22:00): This is a straight-up booty call. (23.00–03.00): Pissed.
Fine.	Not fine. Not at all. You are in the shit.
I'm flirty today, yesterday not, tomorrow?	Mixed signals can reflect stress/indecision – or a calculated way of unsettling you. Either way, play it friendly and cool.
Busy today, maybe another time?	Unless the other time is specified, the 'maybe' is a giveaway. It's a no.
Sorry, missed yr text/didn't check phone/etc	Yeah right.
Tonight? Not sure, will get back to you.	Keeping my options open. You're on the list, but not super high up.
Hey.	I am not the most original texter ever. But I'm into you enough that I texted even though I had nothing to say, so that's cool.

that the feeling you are experiencing is about wanting things to change, rather than to end.

It makes sense to unfriend or block a recent ex on social media, and may spare you some drama. However, don't update your status to 'single' until it is actually true, and don't be surprised if they keep tabs on you via mutual friends.

If it really is the end of the road, have a reason you can communicate. Write something down if it helps focus your thoughts. There is no good argument for leaving someone to waste time wondering what they did wrong when they didn't. Don't get personal, or blamey. Make it be about the

two of you, the something in the dynamic that wasn't quite right, and be prepared to go with a less cheesy version of 'It's not you, it's me'. No one can argue with 'I fell out of love' (though be aware that sometimes 'falling out of love' may just mean you weren't ready to face reality).

Be prepared to take the blame, and maybe some abuse too. If you are leaving them for someone else, you can guarantee they will find out – if that is the case, it might be better just to tell them yourself. Once you've said the words, don't bend – if you aren't going to change your mind, it's cruel to suggest you might. And do not sleep with them. Seriously. Because you will pay for that good time.

LETS TALK ABOUT SEX

I know, you don't need any advice on sex. You're a roving Casanova, who leaves a trail of satisfied lovers in his wake. You can skip this. It isn't for you. This bit is for those other guys. You know. Those looking to improve technique. The ones whose understanding of women's bodies is based on what they've seen in certain online material. The guys who would like to be sure they are making their partner happy, and those who fear they might not make the grade.

Worries

Men worry about sex, but are unlikely to do much about it, other than start worrying about worrying. Which makes it worse. And because it isn't the stuff men talk about with other men, they assume they are the only ones to have concerns. That everyone else is sailing through the bed sheets without a care in the world or a hang-up to call their own. Not so.

Penis size/shape

The most pointless and prevalent of male concerns. Newsflash – there is no standard size or shape. True, to some prospective partners, this matters – but to many, many others, it doesn't. Whatever you have is what you have, which means your only option is to accept it, learn to use it, and keep it clean.

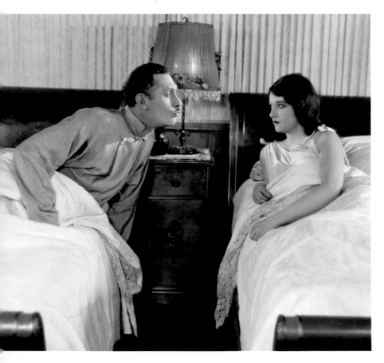

Low sex drive

In a hyper-sexualised world, the man (or woman) who doesn't feel particularly bothered about sex can feel isolated. A low libido can reflect an underlying medical problem – or relationship issues. Or it could be that this is how you are. Whether this is an issue depends entirely on whether it is having a negative effect on your life. If it is, a counsellor or GP can help you understand whether this stems from the physical or the emotional – common causes include tiredness, depression, other sexual problems, or an underlying issue with the relationship.

Impotence

Beer, tiredness, stress – any man who claims he has never experienced the sensation of trying to play snooker with a rope is fibbing. Occasional is one thing, but if this is happening regularly, ignoring it will not help. Causes can be physical (alcohol, smoking, high blood pressure, diabetes) or psychological (stress, anxiety). As with a low sex drive, begin by talking to your GP, who can help you determine whether this is a physical issue that can be addressed with changes to your lifestyle. If you have a partner, counselling together might help.

Premature ejaculation

Some men have the magic and unhelpful ability to go off within seconds of receiving any attention. It may stem from a physical issue, or from anxiety – especially if you are in a new relationship, or otherwise concerned about your performance. If this is you, don't stress it – there are a million techniques to keep it under control. Try masturbating a couple of hours before sex, using an extra-thick condom to reduce sensitivity, or learning techniques to allow you to pause and slow things down. Taking a deep breath at the right moment can postpone the ejaculatory reflex, as can taking a break, or thinking deeply unsexy thoughts. If you have a partner, couples therapy works.

STDs

There's a whole world of nasty bugs out there just waiting to lodge themselves in your privates. Avoidance is better than cure – wear a condom, or regret it. If you need encouragement on this point, leaf through the leaflets at the sexual health clinic, or borrow a baby for the afternoon. If you do find some unexpected itching, spots, or other symptoms down below, get them treated ASAP. If you think you have something, or might have infected someone, the only decent course is honesty. See p102 for more on STDS.

Porn

Where once a man had to shamefacedly smuggle a top-shelf magazine home hidden up his cardigan, now he can access pictures of naked people from the comfort of his own home. It's unlikely mankind will ever give up on porn, despite the many arguments against it – but be aware that constant exposure can have a corrosive effect. If you find your reaction is less than healthy, if it becomes an addiction, if it causes you to have unrealistic expectations of yourself, or others, take a break. PS imitating men in porn films will not go over well in the real world. Because that's fake sex, which people are being paid to do, and wo/men generally want more than a fake plumber who is a pounding pile of muscles. They'd probably prefer a real plumber, who could fix the dripping tap.

Masturbation

As you may have noticed by now, masturbation is not going to make your palms hairy. It is only a health concern if you truly can't stop doing it. It's normal, it's healthy, but there's a time and place.

Virginity

There is no perfect age to lose your virginity, and there are strong arguments against doing it too young. Nevertheless, men who haven't had sex at the point they feel they were 'supposed to' can feel trapped, hopeless, like they have permanently missed the boat. They may also feel unable to discuss it, which makes things worse. If that's you, be aware that despite what you might believe, no one knows. Don't let it define you, and don't let it make you crazy. It will come, and the weird thing is you will be exactly the same guy afterwards.

'Sex without love is as hollow and ridiculous as love without sex'

Hunter S Thompson

How to do sex

There are thousands of sex manuals out there, and this isn't the time or place to give you specific instructions. That said, there are a few rules of thumb that are worth following if you want to have, and give, a good time:

- ◆ Wear a condom, always. Life is too short.
- ◆ Learn the rules of sexual conduct, and respect them and your partner. No means no, always.
- ◆ Practise makes perfect. Not everyone is suited to the experience of multiple partners, but the truth is that playing about a bit does teach you about the world and how to make someone happy. If that isn't you, be cool with it – this is not a competition and you can learn a lot about yourself from masturbation.
- ◆ You can never, ever have enough foreplay. Women may take more time to come to the boil than men – gentle and sensitive holding and kissing will get her there quicker than brisk rubbing. Take your time.
- ◆ Learn about women's bodies, ideally from a woman – if you are straight. There are more erogenous zones at play than the obvious ones – focus on under-appreciated parts, such as the neck. Running your hand over her body will give you a clue. Know where the clitoris is, and how to approach it (slowly, with loving care). If you don't know what and where the G-spot is, Google it.
- ◆ Oral sex is a two-way street. Many women can't orgasm from penetration alone. Don't just learn how to do it – enjoy doing it. If you love your work, it will show.
- ◆ Naked people are vulnerable. Let your partner know s/he is beautiful, and the effect that's having on you.
- ◆ Focus on your partner's needs. Aim to ensure they climax first – and if not, at least don't be the guy that gets his fun and rolls over to sleep.
- ◆ Don't grill your partner on what s/he did or didn't experience. Generally, if you have to ask, they didn't come, but that might not be the end of the world. Talk it through, but don't apply pressure.
- ◆ Never, ever, compare yourself to other guys, or ask how 'X' was in bed.

THE NEXT STEP

There comes a point in every new relationship where one of you asks the big question that's been hovering in the background – what's actually going on here? Are we going to get serious, or call it a day? If you've been drifting along, enjoying the ride, the question may come as a rude surprise. And it is just the first of the many bridges you will have to cross – or burn – together.

What's going on?

You can of course duck the conversation and attempt to extend the honeymoon period, that blissful state where nothing matters but your ability to bring each other fun. When you've reached the point where one of you wants more – security, definition, commitment – it's time for the other to decide if that's what they want too.

If you have different ideas about the future, now is the time to find out. If they are seeing other people and you aren't, if you want kids and they don't, if they want marriage and you want to move to Alaska and become an ice-road trucker, you're both better off knowing, sooner rather than later.

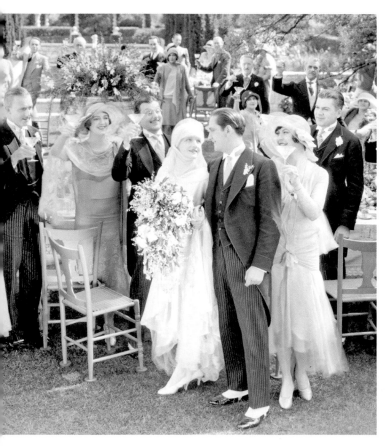

Men and doubt

Doubt is a part of life. If you are feeling uncertain about a relationship shift, don't assume it means you're doing the wrong thing and run off to join the circus. Sometimes even the right course can give a man a bad case of butterflies in the gut. Delaying life changes until you find certainty or perfection will mean a very long wait – possibly the rest of your life. If this relationship is nearly but not quite what you thought you wanted, ask yourself how important the missing bits are before you chuck it over. Equally, if there is a little voice in the back of your head, telling you something about this is not right … listen to it.

Relationship milestones

There's no golden rule for when (or if) you should hit those key moments that say a relationship is moving forwards. What matters is that you are on the same page – if neither of you sees marriage, or a mortgage, or a cat, as a significant part of your love story, then no harm is done by not ticking those boxes. Equally, it is not necessarily harmful to reach these points sooner than you expected.

Cohabitation

The decision to live together is often a mix of practical and romantic considerations, and at some point you'll make it. Probably under time and money pressures.

It is very tempting to make this call on purely pragmatic grounds – accommodation is stressful and expensive, so cohabitation can look like an easy, cheap solution. Beware simple answers to complex problems, though, particularly when a relationship is in its early days. A love based on convenience may not have staying power, and if it ends, one or both of you will have to find somewhere else to live.

Good reasons to move in together include:
◆ you love each other and love each other's company
◆ you're round each other's six nights a week anyway
◆ you are planning a life together
◆ you want to take this to the next stage.

Relationship milestones

Some people may not take this list in this order, which is also cool – though maybe don't contemplate putting number 8 before number 1.

1 Kissing/making out (if the kissing chemistry isn't there, the other stuff won't be either)
2 Sex (when depends on a number of factors, only some of which are in your control – be cool, and don't push it)
3 Holding hands (strangely, this expression of intimacy may only happen after you bump genitals)
4 Introduction to best friends (things are going well, provided they approve of you)
5 Deleting dating apps (if things are going very well, don't keep someone else around as a back-up)
6 Saying 'I love you' (someone has to say it first – if that's you, be cool with the fact they may not feel ready to say it back)
7 First big row (some couples say they don't fight, but they are lying – either to each other, or the rest of us)
8 Updating relationship status (this is you coming out as not single to everyone who knows both of you – for the love of God don't fudge with 'it's complicated' or similar)
9 Binge-watching TV box-sets together (quality sofa time is as important to a relationship as anything bedroom related)

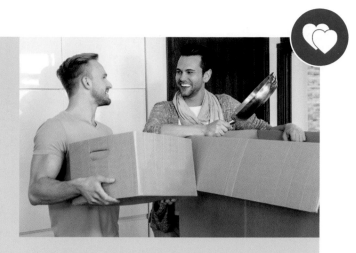

10 Introduction to family (limiting the number of partners you introduce will save you from the helpful feedback of well-meaning relatives who 'always liked that blonde girl, what was her name?')
11 Leave spare stuff at their house (this is you claiming part of the space, like a dog marking territory, but with a toothbrush instead of urine)
12 Referring to them as girlfriend/partner/boyfriend/ whatever (congratulations man, you're a couple)
13 Go on holiday together
14 Move in together (see cohabitation section on p158)
15 Get mortgaged (lower down the order than marriage, despite being more terrifying and more expensive)
16 Get engaged (see popping the question on p160)
17 Get married
18 Breed (if one or both of you isn't into having kids, you will hopefully have established this early on).

Bad reasons to move in together include:
◆ cheaper rent
◆ it might help us get on better/stop fighting
◆ this will really show my ex what they missed out on
◆ their place is really convenient for work
◆ they asked, and I don't want to seem rude.

Before you commit, dry run it. Holidays together are a good dress rehearsal, though be aware that real life isn't beaches and sangria. Spend a week (at least) in the same home, with no breaks for a quick run back to yours. Check their habits – and yours. This is reality, and in reality sometimes lovely people do disgusting things.

My place or yours?
Moving in to theirs, or moving them into yours, may be the easy answer, but be aware that it is someone's zone, and people can be funny about their space. If it is feasible, getting a place together that's new to both of you may be a better place to start.

You will need ground rules, based on ruthless honesty. There is no hiding behind politeness when you share a space, and sucking things up/pretending they don't bother you will not work in the long run. Both of you will have some non-negotiables – equal washing-up duties, no fingernail clipping in the bedroom, etc. Work out the boring but vital stuff in advance about rent/mortgage, bills, etc so that everyone knows what is expected of them.

'Do not let your bachelor ways crystallise, so that you can't soften them when you come to have a wife and family of your own'
Rutherford B Hayes

POPPING THE QUESTION

This is the big one. Bigger, even, than a mortgage application. This is the moment where you finally express the thought that you have found the person you want to be with, forever.

Check yourself

Forever is a long time, so men do not tend to jump into this without some thought. However, if you know from experience that you are the kind of guy who gets carried away easily, it's worth taking some time to reflect on your feelings, and any doubts you may have. Take the same amount of time and care about proposing that you would on deciding about a significant tattoo. On your forehead. Marriage is how you celebrate having found the person you can be with for the rest of your life. It isn't how you fix a relationship that's going wrong, or recover from having been dumped.

Testing the waters

If they've hinted, or flat-out asked, you will know what the answer is before you ask, so the only real question is how you do it. If you aren't sure, test the waters. It's hard to row back from a 'no', so you want to be going into this with as much certainty as possible. Have the big chat about the future and how you both see it. If necessary, ask their friends how they think it will go over – though be ready for them to leak the surprise. The traditional concept of asking her father permission first is now out-dated and straight-out sexist – however, if her family are very formal, consider it a gesture of good faith.

Taking the plunge

Getting the setting right creates a beautiful memory. Think of a proposal plan that reflects how you met, the things you both love to do, your history. Take them to the first place you kissed, the first date venue, your favourite restaurant. Putting some thought and effort into it shows you to be the kind of man anyone would be happy to marry. Be wary of getting over-elaborate – check the plan with a mutual friend for their view on how it might go down, and the random factors that might disrupt your careful scheme.

Many men like a grand gesture – like an engagement proposal in a stadium before kick-off, in front of 40,000 strangers, or a party with everyone either of you have ever known. If you think that is what your partner wants, go for it. Many partners may prefer a little privacy, the sense that this is between you two, and may not enjoy the pressure of all those eyes on them. If your other half is shy, keep it a little more discreet.

If you want to say something about how you feel and why you are asking, write it down, learn it. Don't make it too long – focus on your memories, your feelings, the reasons why you are asking. What about this person makes them the one? When did you first realise that? The longer a speech is, the more opportunity there is to balls it up, so don't make it a drawn-out affair. 'Will you marry me?' usually does the trick.

Whatever you do, and wherever you do it, go down on one knee. There is no other way. It's classy, it shows respect and it's as close as you are ever likely to come to playing a Disney Prince. Dress nice, and maybe have a photographer friend around to record the moment.

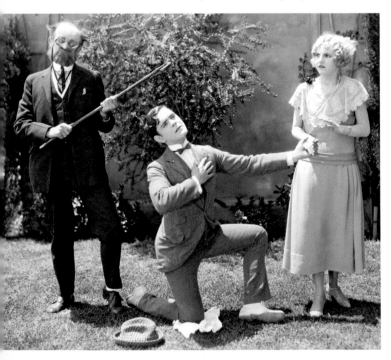

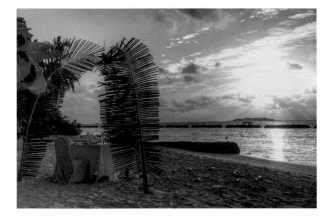

The ring

The ring can be whatever you want it to be, within reason. Traditionally that means a diamond on a slim band, but if funds don't allow, you can always find another way until they do – what is important here is the symbolic declaration of love and commitment, not the money spent. Learn about diamonds, and how they are priced according to Carat, Clarity, Colour and Cut. Choose the jewel in person, from a reputable jeweller – doing your homework will ensure you get the most 'fire' for your buck. There's a rule about spending two months' salary on an engagement ring, but that rule was created by the diamond industry.

There are multiple variables at play with the ring – the metal, which can be white gold, rose gold, yellow gold, platinum – and the setting, or how it sits on (or in) the ring. Unless you are certain you know the taste of your beloved, you may be best off involving them in this process. A good compromise is to buy the diamond and let your partner choose the setting/ring. Or throw caution to the winds and use your best judgement. Do as much research as you can, look at their current jewellery (traditional or modern? Gold, platinum?) and ask mutual friends before you make the call. If you have ninja skills and a ring-sizer, you can check finger size while they sleep.

Wedding plans

How involved you are in plans for the wedding is up to you. Just kidding. It's up to your partner. If you are marrying a woman, the clichéd assumption is generally that this is her big day, and she will have an idea of how she wants it to go. If that's the case, your main role is support, doing whatever is needed doing to help it run smoothly. If it's more of a team effort, then you need to come to a shared understanding of what you want, how much it will cost, and who is paying (guys marrying guys may lean towards this more collegiate approach).

Either way, your input is going to be vital in at least a few areas, such as the guest list and venue. This is where you cannot avoid having an opinion – which you may be able to get away with on questions about flowers and crockery. The best solution is to go down the long list of things to be organised – the date, the place, the people, the food, the music – and establish between you where your help would be appreciated, and where your best bet would be to shut up and smile.

Stress

It's a hugely stressful time, which can cause you to look at the crazed person who is now your fiancée and wonder whether you are doing the right thing. Make sure you take regular breaks from the planning to enjoy each other's company and focus on more positive stuff. The honeymoon is an obvious candidate – looking for romantic B&Bs on the beach in Costa Rica is significantly more fun than booking an organist. If your honeymoon is months after the ceremony, consider a 'minimoon' just after the wedding.

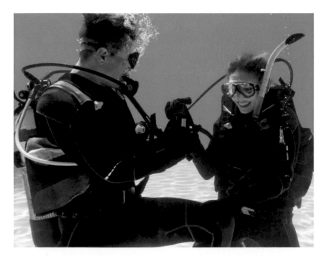

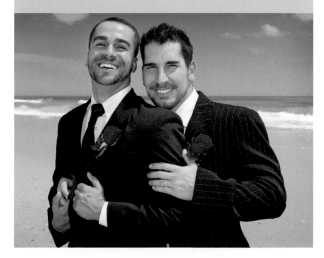

BEING SINGLE

There's a lot of advice available for men who want to be with someone. It's an assumption society makes – that a man can only be happy with a romantic partner. In truth, many people can find themselves perfectly happy alone. And learning to enjoy his own company is probably the best thing any man can do, even when it isn't his ultimate plan. Take some time off the relationship merry-go-round and hang out with yourself.

Dealing with heartbreak

If you've just been dumped, divorced or otherwise let down, bouncing back may not be high on your to-do list. You may instead feel more like drowning yourself in a lake of whisky, howling sorrow at the moon, or desperately pleading for someone to return your love. Those are understandable impulses when you feel like someone has removed your nuts, stuffed them in a sack weighted down with your heart, and thrown it into the canal.

It's OK to wallow in self-pity for a while, to be shell-shocked in response to rejection, and to think of ways you can let them know what an asshole they are. What isn't OK is acting on those thoughts. Do not indulge in any act of love revenge, however much you think it is justified, including any mean-spirited messages you might have been thinking of sending. That just shows your hurt pride and makes you look like a fool. Hurting them will do nothing to make you feel better. The best revenge is to move on and be happy.

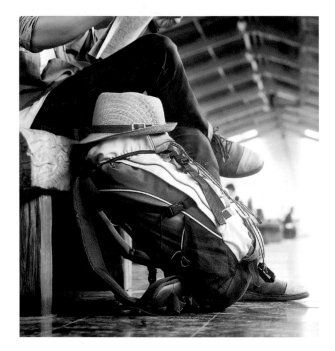

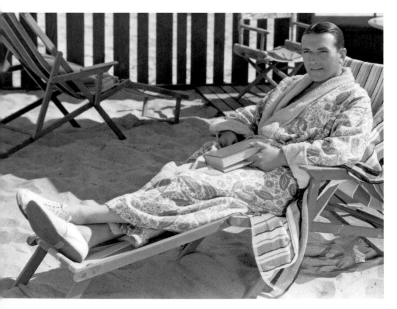

Acceptance

You can't even start to get back to feeling like yourself until you've accepted it's over. Easier said than done, but you have no choice but to try. Let yourself grieve. Bottling it up, sticking a cork in it, soldiering on and pretending there isn't a gaping wound where your heart used to be DOES NOT WORK. Do what you can to let the dark thoughts out of your system. Moan to your friends, until they are bored of hearing it and you are bored of saying it. Write it down, if that helps you process. Be as gutted, as down, as sorrowful as you need to be, but accept that what is done is done, and that nothing you do or say now will change the past.

There is, however, a present and a future to deal with, and both of them will be better, particularly if you can learn something from what just happened. Did it get full-on too fast? Did you put your trust in someone when your judgement told you otherwise? How did how your actions

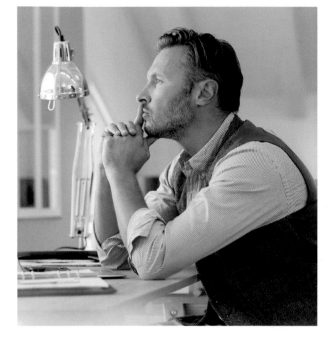

impact the relationship – and what could you do differently next time?

Thinking of the future can take an enormous act of will on your part when it feels like there isn't one. And yet no one knows what happens next. You may feel worthless, but that doesn't mean someone isn't going to fall for you, sooner than you imagine. Remind yourself of your good qualities, the stuff that made your ex fall for you in the first place, the stuff they are now missing out on. The sucker.

Some people will say they can't accept a relationship is over until they've had an answer that makes sense to them. Those people are out of luck. Because an ex is unlikely to say anything that will persuade you it was the right thing for you, and a desire for this kind of 'closure' often means you want the chance to talk them out of it. The only person who can make you feel ready to accept this is you.

Distract yourself. Exercise is good, letting you get rid of the tension and anger in a safe way. Treat your body with care – this is not a time to live off instant noodles and beer. Alcohol is a short-term solution, which only postpones the pain.

If you've tried it all, and you are still struggling to move on, then you may need assistance. Counselling can help you work out if this relates to something else in your life, and figure out what steps you need to take to jump back in the fray.

Alone time

If you've always been with someone and never had a significant period of bachelor time, and the opportunity presents itself, do it. Be alone. Commit to taking yourself off the market for a while. You can define for yourself what that means – no dating, no serious dating, celibacy, or just putting friends first. Whatever rule you create, stick with it and learn to enjoy your own company.

Even if you believe you are ultimately heading for love and marriage and the baby carriage, this down time is a good idea. Because you can't be happy with someone else until you are happy with your own self. Jumping from partner to partner is a way of papering over the cracks, allowing yourself to ignore the issues you cart around. Facing those demons, and dealing with them, will make you ready for love, or whatever else you have in mind.

Being alone gives you time to reflect, recharge and relax. It also means you get to stop compromising. There's no one else to satisfy, no one to apologise to or try to keep happy. You won't have to look to anyone else to give you advice or tell you what you should do next. All those rules about what a partner is looking for, and how to be a grown-up? Ignore them. Leave your pants on the floor, have breakfast for dinner and grow your nose hair. Treat yourself. Take yourself out, do the things you like to do, alone or with others. Have fun.

Learning to enjoy your own company is a gift for life – because whatever else happens, you are going to be spending a long time with yourself. Might as well be sure you get on.

'Outside of a dog, a book is a man's best friend. Inside of a dog it's too dark to read'
Groucho Marx

Postscript

The role of man has changed over time, but the fundamentals remain the same. Stand tall, be your own man, look after others, open doors for people, wear clean socks. Learn how to dance, cook the perfect omelette, pack a suitcase and wear a pocket square. Make sure your home is your castle, your shoes are shiny, and your conscience is clear. Enjoy your own company and listen to others, be the guy who people turn to when the going gets rough and the guy who knows when to ask for help.

If you can do all these things, and more – and you can, because you read the damn book – then, my son, you are a man.

Acknowledgements

Thanks to Andrew Webb (author of the awesome Men's Baking Manual) for making this happen, to Louise at Haynes for bringing me on board and setting this in the right direction, Joanne for her great eye for detail and excellent way with a recipe and Lucy for her light and sensitive touch in making these words better than they deserved to be. Cheers to Dylan Collard, the best portrait photographer in the UK.

A tip of the hat to all who chipped in with thoughts, including but not limited to: Joseph Hart; Murray Healy; Lucy Shaw; and Hossein at Cutter and Grinder, Brighton. What I know about being a man I picked up from friends – Dale, Gerard, Philip, Shadric, Scott, Steve, Stephen, Will, George, Martin and Jem – and family – Maurice Hargreaves, Mike Knowles, Giovanni Baglione and John Hutt have all been men to look up to and learn from. I wouldn't have been able to write a book about men if I hadn't spent so much time listening to the wise words of women – thank you Geraldine, Jennifer, Liza, Janet and most of all Catherine Hargreaves.

This book wouldn't have been half as good without Francesca's insight and love, and neither would I. Luciana is the most awesome kid in the world, so this is for her.